OBESITY EXPLOSION

THE COLLISION OF NUTRITION, CULTURE, POLITICS & FOOD

[JOSEPH LEONARD DIXON, PH.D.]

Kendall Hunt
publishing company

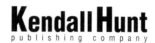

CONTENTS

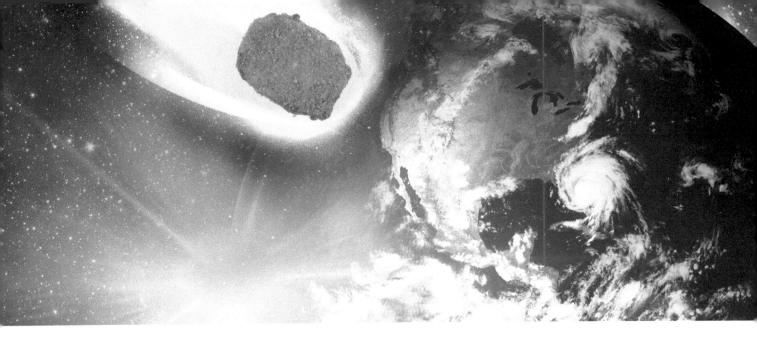

PART 1

Introduction—The Mystery of Obesity—When Did Obesity Explosion Occur?

Where Did Obesity Come From?

Why is there obesity? What happened to Americans such that two out of three of adults are overweight or obese? Did our genetics suddenly go crazy all of a sudden? Maybe Aliens visited and targeted humans and made us too immobile to fight back?

Whatever the reasons are for the Obesity Explosion, they must be powerful, because after hundreds of thousands of years as Hunter—Gatherers, and 10,000 years of living and striving in a largely agriculture-based world, we have morphed into creatures beings that carry around extra energy, that is, obese creatures.

The answers for what caused obesity are out there, but they are just really hard to see. There is a great amount of misinformation out there, too—especially coming from the "pseudonutrition experts," who are, in fact, not experts, but people who deal in pseudoscience. They use terms that sound correct, but their reasoning and facts are anything but correct. And, of course, misinformation has been multiplied by social media. Welcome to the new world.

I have been teaching a class called Nutrition and Health for over 25 years. It has taken me 3 years to write this book, but I have been preparing it for 25 years. I wrote this book because there are only a few good nutrition books designed for the curious nonscientific mind. There are plenty of textbooks for college students and researchers, but none that are focused and specifically designed to tell the whole story of obesity in our everyday lives.

My goal for this book is if people really understood what was involved in nutrition and health, they wouldn't fall for all the misinformation out there. They might feel better about themselves because they would be confident that they were following accurate and truthful advice. In doing so, they could get a glimpse of the wonder of it all—the way nutrition and our bodies really work. And it is not that hard!

My thesis is that on the whole, the Obesity Explosion in America resulted from monumental eruptions in the ways life changed in America. Some of these changing life factors we can see (as in more conveniences), and there are some that we can't easily see (as in the development of new foods). Some factors are under a person's control, and some factors are difficult for anyone to control. After reading this book, you will see that for most of us, the most potent way to combat obesity is to change both our lifestyle and what we eat. I know that unless people really see a logical and meaningful way to maintain health, they are not going to give up important conveniences or change their life. At the same time, I can't let "internet nutrition experts," who know very little about nutrition, blame individual things such as sugar or certain fats. Their gullible followers are made to believe that if they change that one single thing, it will solve their weight and happiness problems. People who have tried many crackpot solutions, and who have failed multiple times with them, go on to develop a feeling of hopelessness (discussed in depth in a later chapter). Eventually, they stop doing anything concerning their health. Why bother?

So where does this book take you? There are no easy fixes presented in this book. And it may possibly take you to places you have never been to. And yes, there is some science in this book. You may be able to skip over some of it. I hope you will plow through the science. In the end it will help you understand.

So let's go to the problem first.

The Obesity Explosion erupted in the late 1970s, with 1980 being the year where we could see a verifiable upturn in the rates of obesity. But what lit the fuse of the proverbial obesity bomb that blew up the regulation systems that had maintained body weight in humans for over 20,000 years? Certainly there are no reports of obesity during the 10,000 years of agriculture. Something happened, but what was it? We will travel through a good deal of time—back several hundred years ago and up to the present time. We will eventually travel to the precise year obesity took off, and examine what I believe ignited the obesity bomb. But who lit the fuse? And why? I will attempt to answer these questions.

The Obesity Explosion and its causes remind me of the cataclysmic killing off of the dinosaurs, and many other species, 66 million years ago. A 10-kilometer-wide meteoroid hit the Earth, and the dinosaurs just did not have time to adapt and survive when that fateful day arrived. Although humans have had a little more time, we have not yet adapted to the changes in food and lifestyles that occurred in the past 50 years.

As theoretical particle physicist, Lisa Randall discussed in her extraordinary book, *Dark Matter and the Dinosaurs*[1]:

---

[1] Randall L. (2015). *Dark Matter and the Dinosaurs. The Astounding Interconnectedness of the Universe*. New York: HarperCollins Publishers. Ecco Imprint, Introduction, page xiv.

"Natural selection permits adaptation when species have time to evolve. But the adaptation won't encompass radical changes. It is far too slow. The dinosaurs weren't in a position to prepare for a 10-kilometer-wide meteoroid hitting the Earth. They couldn't adapt. Those stuck on land, who were too big to bury themselves, had nowhere viable to go."

Just like the dinosaurs, humans have not adapted to the life-altering changes that shook the way we lived in the 1900s. But it is not a time issue. It is more of a knowledge issue.

But what seems like a very straightforward problem turns out not to be so simple after a little investigation.

Humans survived, multiplied, and spread across the Earth because they were able to adapt to almost every environment and food source. Adaptability in humans was made possible due to a brain that could learn quickly and forge solutions to unique problems. The success of humankind has led to a total Earth population of more than seven billion people, a remarkable number that dwarfs the 1,500 people that survived at Pinnacle Point, South Africa, possibly where modern humans developed during the last great ice age of 200,000 years ago.[2]

The story concerning obesity fills only a short, recent, 50-year period. A failure to adapt caused the current widespread accumulation of excess body energy in the form of fat, which, in aggregate, I call the Obesity Explosion. From what we know of human history, with its twists and turns, this crisis will surely abate when the availability of food becomes scarce due to climate change, or depletion of soil nutrients, or due to a pandemic. But in the meantime, the Obesity Explosion will be with us for some time to come, and the reasons for this shift in humankind are the subject of this book.

---

[2] Marean CW (2010). When the sea saved humanity. *Sci Am* 303(2): 53–61 (August). http://www.ncbi.nlm.nih.gov/pubmed/?term=PMID%3A+++++20684373

What is Obesity and When did the Obesity Explosion Start in the U.S.?

In the previous chapter I mentioned that something catastrophic had occurred in our country (and throughout the world) that caused the Obesity Explosion. But what was it? In order to define what happened, and define what caused the Obesity Explosion, we have to know how to define obesity. Yes, it is extra body energy, that is, extra weight. But what is the very best way to identify and study it? Humans come in all shapes and sizes. Some are small and some are large. Some have frail bones, and some have big, heavy bones. Some have short legs, and others have extremely long legs. Some people have very slight muscles, and some are muscular all over. How can all these different types of people be measured and categorized in an experimentally usable way?

What Is the Official Definition of Obesity?

For most of the 1900s, body weights were categorized using tables developed by actuaries at Insurance Companies. Little is known about how these tables were constructed or who even developed them. Body weight alone is not adequate because of the vast spectrum of heights in humans. Since then, scientists have sought to develop a metric that can be used in studies to stratify human body weights into distinct groups. At the current time, most scientists and physicians use the Body Mass Index, or BMI, which adjusts an adult's body weight (in kilograms) for their height (converted to meters squared). The calculation (for both sexes) is:

$$\text{BMI} = \text{body weight in kilograms}/(\text{height in meters})^2$$

The best way to calculate BMI is to go to the Centers for Disease Control (CDC) website[1] and use their BMI calculator. For children there is a different way to evaluate obesity, and this is explained on the CDC website, too.

For Americans who feel more comfortable with pounds and inches (and that includes me too) there is a way to convert the original definition equation to pounds and inches, and it is shown below:

BMI Calculations with Pounds and Inches

$$\text{Body Mass Index} = \frac{\text{Weight}(\text{Pounds})}{\text{Height}(\text{Inches})^2} \times 703 =$$

For a 5 ft, 6 in tall person (66 in tall); BMI changes with weight as follows:

Weight		BMI	
112 lb	$\text{Body Mass Index} = \dfrac{\text{Weight}(112)}{\text{Height}(66)^2} \times 703 =$	18.1	underweight
124 lb		20	normal
136 lb		22	
155 lb		25	overweight
173 lb		28	
186 lb		30	obese
198 lb		32	

Therefore, using this equation with a conversion factor allows you to calculate your BMI easily using pounds and inches. But still the easiest way is to Google "CDC BMI Calculator," and the correct page from the CDC will show up in the search list.

Below is a table from the CDC explaining what the BMI categories stand for.

---

[1] https://www.cdc.gov/healthyweight/assessing/bmi/

How is BMI interpreted for adults?

For adults 20 years old and older, BMI is interpreted using standard weight status categories. These categories are the same for men and women of all body types and ages.

The standard weight status categories associated with BMI ranges for adults are shown in the following table.

BMI	Weight Status
Below 18.5	Underweight
18.5–24.9	Normal or Healthy Weight
25.0–29.9	Overweight
30.0 and Above	Obese

It must be stated that BMI is not a foolproof way to denote obesity levels. In fact, BMI is not by itself a definitive way to determine body fatness or the health of an individual. "In general, BMI is an inexpensive and easy-to-perform method of screening for weight category, for example, underweight, normal or healthy weight, overweight, and obesity." The biggest difficulty is with highly muscular people who tend to have high BMIs without the level of fat that is considered obese. Very muscular people will be quite heavier than average, and therefore their BMI will calculate to be on the high side. A famous example is calculating the BMI of Arnold Schwarzenegger when he was a committed weight lifter. Putting his values (240 lb; 6 ft 2 in height) into the BMI calculator, you come up with a BMI of 30.8, which would indicate that Arnold was obese at the time. However, if you told him this to his face, he might show you personally that he is, in fact, not obese. I myself would not be brave enough to tell Arnold Schwarzenegger face to face he was obese!!

The following two graphs illustrate how imperfect BMI is when evaluating individuals. In the first graph, I show an approximation of the relationship between BMI and percent body fat in men. The Trend line in blue shows the relationship closely similar to the real relationship. The hypothetical observations in orange triangles would be how observations of individual people in a research study would cluster closely around the Trend line if the relationship between BMI and percent body fat was precise and accurate.

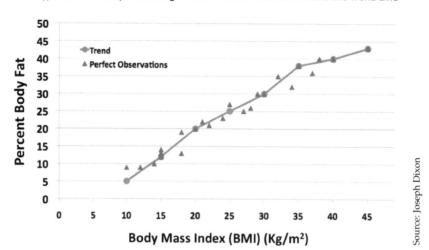

Hypothetical Example Showing if Observations Clustered Around the Trend Line

Source: Joseph Dixon

However, this is not the case at all. Below is from an actual study and the graph charts calculated BMI versus percent body fat in men as measured by the dual-energy X-ray absorptiometry (DEXA) method.[2] The data for this study were taken from the National Health and Nutrition Examination Survey (NHANES). This is a program that studies the health and nutritional status of adults and children in the United States.[3] In this particular arm of the study, the scientists measured percent body fat by using DEXA. When the data for measured percent body weight are plotted versus BMI, you can see that there is wide variation in percent body fat for men of the same BMI. The drawn curvilinear line on the graph below is the best-fit regression curve and explains the distribution of values for the population taken as a whole.

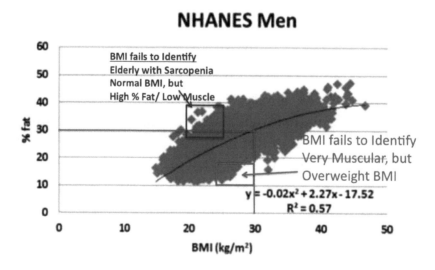

NHANES Men

---

[2] Gonzalez MC, Correia MITD, Heymsfield SB (2017). A requiem for BMI in the clinical setting. *Curr Opin Clin Nutr Metab Care* 20(5):314–321. https://www.ncbi.nlm.nih.gov/pubmed/28768291. This is a section from Figure 1. Important quote in the paper: "This observation shows that BMI has a limited predictive value at the individual level."

[3] https://www.cdc.gov/nchs/nhanes/about_nhanes.htm

For example, a man with a BMI of 30 (red vertical line) could have a percent body fat anywhere between 18% and 40%. No doubt, Arnold Schwarzenegger had a body fat content below 20% even though his BMI was over 30. Also, one can see that some men (inside the blue-lined box) have very high percent body fat, but their measurements would calculate to a healthy BMI (between 18.5 and 24.9). This group would include older men who have sarcopenia (loss of lean muscle mass). So, having little muscle and lots of fat could translate into a healthy BMI.

It would definitely be better to perform a direct measurement of body fat during regular examinations. But this is a very expensive test to do in a large population. However, routine percent body fat measurements may one day become a reality.

Even in times before the current problem with weight gain, 4% to 6% of individuals in the population were considered heavy (I am using the term heavy because this was before BMI came into use). The reason for this small percentage of heavy people is that for every biological function in humans, there is a wide range of responses that make people different from their neighbors. And one of these responses that can vary widely is the efficient accumulation of energy in the face of low food availability. The presence of a segment of people that was very efficient in gaining and holding on to extra energy meant that there would be individuals in the group, village, or tribe, who would survive the next famine and keep the group going. And because women were more important to repopulate the tribe, it made evolutionary sense that most heavy individuals were women.

But what about the present—specifically the past 40 to 50 years? Why has America gone through an unprecedented increase in obesity in this country? We have tons of data on what happened, but we don't know why it happened. That is what this book is about—why it happened. Let's look at the most basic data on this topic. Here is a pertinent quote:[4]

> "Analysis of the National Health and Nutrition Examination Survey (NHANES) data suggests that the average daily energy intake increased from 1971 to 2000. The average increase was 168 kcal/day for men and 335 kcal/day for women. With no active regulation or adaptation of energy balance, this increase theoretically could explain a yearly weight gain of 18 lb for men and 35 lb for women."

So there is no doubt that Americans are eating more on a daily basis, and by energy considerations alone, the increase in weight should be even greater than what has been observed in the American public over the past 50 years. Therefore, Americans have adapted a little, and they have tried to resist gaining weight, but the very

---

[4] Hill JO, Wyatt HR, Peters JC (2012). Energy balance and obesity. *Circulation* 126(1): 126–132. http://www.ncbi.nlm.nih.gov/pubmed/22753534

complex food intake regulation system that is present in each of us has not been able to fully contain the onslaught of many factors ("Death by a thousand paper cuts") that have confronted us in the past 50 years.

When Did the Obesity Explosion Start?

Now that we know how to define obesity, let's look at the changes in the obesity rates in the United States over the past 50 years. In later chapters, we will look closer at changes in the consumption of foods that occurred during this same period.

The increase in obesity in the US is shown in the next series of figures:

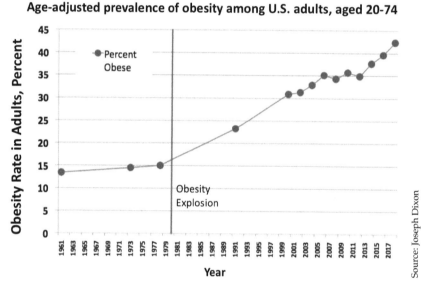

Data for this graph are from various U.S. Government studies as described in the reports referenced below. The red vertical line at 1980 I denote as the Obesity Explosion.

The above data from the NHANES[5] shows the rise in obesity rate in adults from 1961 to around 2017, when the increase appeared to halt. Additional data has indicated that the prevalence of obesity in adults is still increasing such that in

---

[5] NOTE from the CDC: Estimates for adults aged 20 and over were age adjusted by the direct method to the 2000 U.S. Census population. Earlier Data: Prevalence of Overweight, Obesity, and Extreme Obesity Among Adults: United States, Trends 1960–1962 Through 2007–2008 by Cynthia L. Ogden, Ph.D., and Margaret D. Carroll, M.S.P.H., Division of Health and Nutrition Examination Surveys, June 2010; Later data: Trends in age-adjusted obesity and severe obesity prevalence among adults aged 20 and over: United States, 1999–2000 through 2017–2018. SOURCE: NCHS, National Health and Nutrition Examination Survey; NCHS Data Brief No. 360, February 2020. https://www.cdc.gov/nchs/products/databriefs/db360.htm

2013–2014 the percent was 37.7%, and in 2015–2016, the percent shot up to 39.6% of adults were classified as obese.[6]

The graph shows that by 2007 roughly one third of Americans were characterized as obese (BMI ≥30 kg/m^2). The graph starts at 1961 because the NHANES studies started just prior to this date. In fact, there is only weak data on percent obesity for the time periods earlier than this (possibly because it was not recognized as a problem before this time). If you use data from small studies, the trend line prior to 1961 would slowly become rather flat and would level off at around 4% to 5% of the population in the period around the year 1900. On the above graph, the trend line shows what appears to be a steady increase from 1978 to 1980 to around 2010, but there are, in fact, differences in the slopes of the component lines, and these differences are hard to discern. Therefore, I regraphed the data for the obesity rate as percent increase per year in between the surveys. Although this analysis suffers from different lengths of the periods between the surveys, basing it per year should alleviate misinterpretations. The graph shows that there were relatively small increases between the first surveys, and then there is a fantastic increase between the 1980 and 1994 surveys. Also, there were large increases thereafter, with the greatest percent increase per year occurring between the 1994 and 2000 surveys. This presentation of the data leads to the unmistakable conclusion that something happened in the period around 1980, or in the 10-year period prior to 1980, that disrupted the ability of humans to adapt to a change in their environment. In most of the graphs in this book, I have drawn a vertical red line at or around the year 1980 to mark this observation.

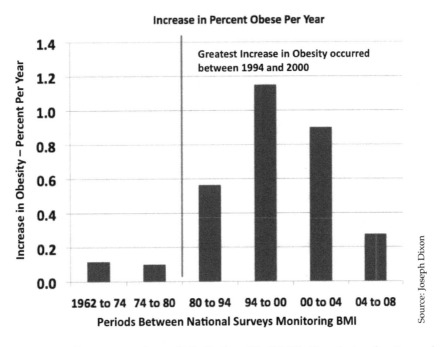

[6] Hales CM, Fryar CD, Carroll MD, Freedman DS, Ogden CL (2018). Trends in obesity and severe obesity prevalence in US youth and adults by sex and age, 2007–2008 to 2015–2016. *JAMA* (16):1723–1725. https://pubmed.ncbi.nlm.nih.gov/29570750

The next graph splits the data (now presented as average BMI) for men and women in order to discern whether there were differences in the responses of men and women to the period around and following 1980. The graph clearly shows, and the results are really quite amazing, that both men and women responded in equivalent ways to whatever happened around the year 1980, or the period immediately before it. Considering how different men and women are in terms of basal metabolic rates, hormone profiles, and activity levels during the day, the fact that both groups responded similarly in gaining BMI is shocking. Something absolutely powerful must have occurred during this period in order to increase BMI similarly in men and women.

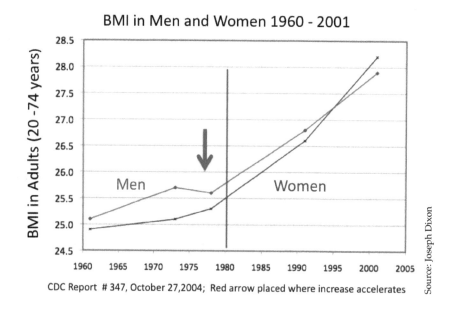

CDC Report # 347, October 27, 2004; Red arrow placed where increase accelerates

The previous graphs were for adults. What is the situation in children? Below is a graph of prevalence of overweight (including obese) children in a group of countries over the period from 1974 to around 2005.[7] Just as with adults, the prevalence increased in children during the same period.

Very disturbing is that, when the data of overweight and obese children are examined across several countries (including developed and developing countries), the United States leads in children being overweight and obese. The children in the U.S. start off at 15% overweight and obese and end up at 35% by 2004. The smallest increase in obesity was observed in Japan.

---

[7] Swinburn BA, Sacks G, Hall KD, McPherson K, Finegood DT, Moodie ML, Gortmaker SL (2011). The global obesity pandemic: shaped by global drivers and local environments. *Lancet* 378: 804–814. http://www.thelancet.com/journals/lancet/article/PIIS0140-6736%2811%2960813-1/fulltext

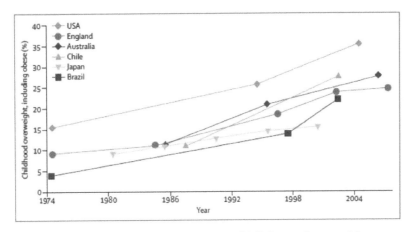

Lancet 2011; 378: 804–14   Children: Age < 18 years

The above graphs should be considered extraordinary when one considers how humans have lived, survived, and adapted to an agricultural way of life over the past 10,000 years. Why did both children and adults have eruptions in obesity starting on or around 1980? What occurred in our society that influenced the increase in obesity similarly in men and women? What circumstances occurred that were able to completely wreak havoc with the finely tuned, biological regulatory mechanism that developed over the past 200,000 years or more to control food intake and body weight in *Homo sapiens*?

These are mysteries of immense proportions because they are closely associated with the health of tens of millions of Americans. Is there one factor that caused the rise in obesity after 10,000 years of agriculture during which obesity was not a problem whatsoever? Or did many factors come together to cause the Obesity Explosion? From the graphs that I have provided, I am going to call 1980 the actual start date of the Obesity Explosion!

I wish to covey the big picture behind why it was so difficult to maintain body weight in the second half of the 20th century, and which continues today. Because only through knowing the entire picture will a true understanding of the Obesity Explosion be achieved, and this knowledge will either make us feel better, make us feel worse, or put us on a more solid footing and allow us to combat in a safe and logical way the misregulation of controlling weight.

In other words, the purpose of this book is to ask:

Why Did the Obesity Explosion Occur?

And follow where all the data points lead to!

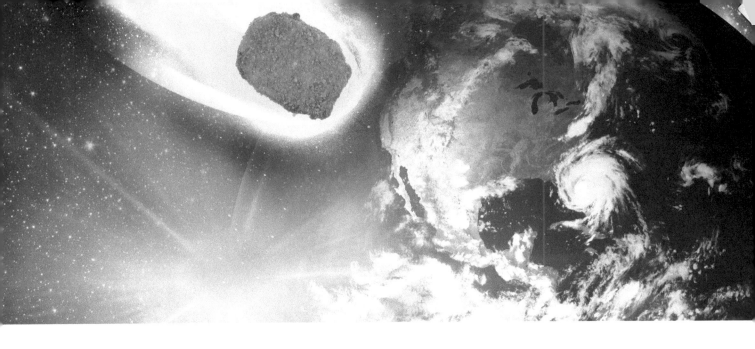

PART 2

Early Humans, Changes to our Food, and Factors that Led to the Obesity Explosion

Ancient Societies—The Dominance of Principal Starches as Food

A recent ancestor to *Homo sapiens* was *Homo erectus*, who lived from two million to 500,000 years ago. During this period of time, the prehuman cranial capacity increased and the intestinal architecture changed to a small stomach/long small intestine structure. It is hypothesized that these changes were linked to the intake of a higher–energy-containing diet. To provide such a diet, it is generally assumed that somewhere during this time Homo erectus began to cook his or her food. The first confirmed use of fire for cooking food is from Qesem Cave in Israel, which contained evidence for cooking around 400,000 years ago. But many authorities believe that cooking started much earlier than this.[1] The premodern humans of the species Homo erectus certainly were most likely mainly gatherers who at some point learned to cook their foods with fire. This allowed for the more efficient digestion of the carbohydrates and other macronutrients in plant foods.[2]

The Life and Diet of Hunter–Gatherers (H-G)

Before agriculture was adopted, humans led a hunter–gatherer existence, a lifestyle that limited the total numbers of humans. There are many excellent reviews of this type of lifestyle and the diets eaten.[3-6]

---

[1] Wrangham R (2009). *Catching Fire: How Cooking Made Us Human.* New York: Basic Books.

[2] Hardy K, Brand-Miller J, Brown KD, Thomas MG, Copeland L (2015). The importance of dietary carbohydrate in human evolution. *Q Rev Biol* 90(3): 251–268. https://www.ncbi.nlm.nih.gov/pubmed/26591850

[3] Levi-Strauss C (English translation with John Weightman, Translator; Doreen Weightman, Translator; Patrick Wilcken, Introduction) (1955). *Tristes Tropiques.* Modern English translation: Penguin Classics Paperback (January 31, 2012).

The take-home points of a wide variety of studies of the lives and diets of terrestrial hunter–gatherers (H-G) in tropical and moderate environments come down to (1) In most cases, H-G worked fewer hours per day to obtain their required calories than early farmers did. (2) H-G needed to move on a continual basis to a new location within their extensive roaming territory in order to find regions that were not depleted of edible plants and animal game. (3) Even though H-G groups were quite small, a large area of land was required to support a roaming band of H-G. (4) There was always the possibility that a drought or a short, cold growing season (for wild plants) would decrease the supply of gatherable food for H-G, leading to starvation and the destruction of the group. In such cases a band would disperse and people would merge with other bands as a survival mechanism.

Humans transitioned to agriculture around 8000–9000 BC. But even before this, humans collected wild grass grains for thousands of years. Societies relied upon agriculture to sustain themselves and enlarge their populations.

New research has been unearthed in the past 20 years indicating that early agriculture and urbanization started at approximately the same time in the Fertile Crescent and on the western coast of South America. Dr. Peter Bellwood has written that "Agriculture emerged as the predominant form of food production directly from a hunter–gatherer background, without any major significant attributable external diffusion, in at least five major regions of the world..."[7] These areas where agriculture spontaneously sprouted include Southwest Asia (the Fertile Crescent); South and Central America; Eastern China near the Yangzi and Yellow Rivers; New Guinea; and the last region to be establish agriculture, the Woodlands of the Eastern United States. Humans collected wild grain long before grains were domesticated, and the practice spread where ever humans went. They gathered wild grass grains in Europe very early after they left Africa. A pestle grinder was discovered in a cave near the village of Paglicci in south eastern Italy, near the Gargano Peninsula. On the grinder were Avena (Avenabarbata) (oat) starch grains that probably were meant for flour preparation. The grinder dated to 32,614 + 429 years before present. This finding, and the others grinders found in diverse areas, shows that the inhabitants

---

[4] Cordain L, Brand-Miller J, Eaton SB, Mann N, Holt SHA, Speth JD (2000). Plant to animal subsistence ratios and macronutrient energy estimations in world-wide hunter–gatherer diets. *Am J Clin Nutr* 71: 682–692. http://ajcn.nutrition.org/content/71/3/682.long

[5] Bellwood P. (2005). *First Farmers: The Origins of Agricultural Societies.* Malden, MA: Blackwell Publishing, see Chapter 2.

[6] Marean CW (2016). The transition to foraging for dense and predictable resources and its impact on the evolution of modern humans. *Phil Trans R Soc B* 371: pii: 20150239. https://www.ncbi.nlm.nih.gov/pubmed/27298470 and http://dx.doi.org/10.1098/rstb.2015.0239

[7] Bellwood P (2005). Ibid, p. 42.

of Europe prepared flour from collected wild grass grains. The determined age of the implements provides evidence for flour preparation much earlier than previously reported.[8]

Wheat was domesticated in the Fertile Crescent approximately 9000–8000 BC. This occurred at several sites, including the village of Abu Hureyra, which contained 5,000 inhabitants at this time.

At about the same period as events unfolded in the Fertile Cresent, marine foods were harvested along the coast of South America at Quebrada Jaguay (11,000 BC). By 8000 BC, beans, squash, and peppers were harvested by humans living in what is now Peru. Cassava and potatoes were domesticated (7000–6000 BC) in the Amazon and Andes regions of South America, respectively. Later, around 5000 BC, maize (corn), was domesticated in the region we now call Mexico, using plant breeding and growing methods that are still being investigated and debated by scientists today. Also around 5000 BC, and on the other side of the Pacific Ocean, rice was domesticated in Eastern China.

Recent Evidence of the Importance of Marine Foods to Humans

Agriculture on land was not the only source of a significant food supply. When anthropologist Dr. Michael E. Moseley traveled to Peru and worked on Peruvian coast sites in 1966–1967, he realized that the maritime population that had lived there was very complex, as he and his colleagues discovered magnificent architectural layouts, including raised platforms, that signaled high social order and complexity. Although the land immediate inland from the Pacific Ocean is bone dry, a coastal current hugs the shore as it flows north, providing the "richest maritime environment in the New World."[9] With these observations in mind, Dr. Moseley wrote, *The Maritime Foundations of Andean Civilization*, a book in which he described his observations and proposed the hypothesis that it was access to marine foods that started the progression to a full human civilization on the western coast of South America.

Dr. Moseley later refined his hypothesis and related how early humans moved to using both marine foods and early farming to obtain a diverse diet.[10] Another early

---

[8] Mariotti LM, Foggi B, Aranguren B, Ronchitelli A, Revedin A (2015). Multistep food plant processing at Grotta Paglicci (Southern Italy) around 32,600 cal B.P. *Proc Natl Acad Sci U S A.* (39): 12075–12080. https://www.ncbi.nlm.nih.gov/pubmed/26351674

[9] Moseley ME (1975). *The Maritime Foundations of Andean Civilization.* Menlo Park, CA: Cummings Publishing Company, p. 9.

[10] Moseley ME (1992). Maritime foundations and multilinear evolution: Retrospect and prospect. *Andean Past* 3: 5–42.

discovery of Dr. Moseley's was his finding of the early cultivation of cotton, which was used for clothing and many other purposes, including woven materials used to formulate fishing nets.[11]

What About Our Current Time?

Although marine foods were important in the rise of major civilizations, the "principal starches" were what fed practically every group of humans throughout the world.

I refer to plant foods enriched with energy-packed complex carbohydrates as "principal starches," which is the term Sidney Mintz used in his book on the history of sugar.[12] My definition of a "principal starch" is in a footnote.[13]

What Was the Role of the Principal Starch in Early Villages?

Dr. Mintz wrote about the role of principal starches in the village[14]:

> People subsist on some principal complex carbohydrate, usually a grain or root crop, around which their lives and villages and small cities are built. Its calendar of growth fits with their calendar of the year; its needs are, in some curious ways, their needs. It provides the raw materials out of which much of the meaning in life is given voice. Its character, names, distinctive tastes and textures, the difficulties associated with its cultivation, its history, mythical or not, are projected on the human affairs of people who consider what they eat to be a basic food, to be *the* definition of food.

The principal starch was processed so as to be digestible and useful in the preparation of meals. The collected grain or root materials were first ground using stones, and later when the technology was improved, using mortars and pestles, and then mixed

---

[11] Stephens SG, Moseley ME (1973). Cotton remains from archaeological sites in Central Coastal Peru. *Science* 180: 186–188.

[12] Mintz SW (1985). *Sweetness and Power: The Place of Sugar in Modern History.* New York: Penguin Books, p. 10.

[13] A "principal starch" in most societies was a hand manipulated, stone ground food made from plants such as wheat, corn, or a root crop (tuber) that contained the two major forms of complex carbohydrates-starch, which is digestible and provides glucose for energy, and fiber, which is indigestible and does not provide energy to humans. In most cases, the stone processed foods, which still needed to be cooked, resulted in a mixture that contained, by weight, an average of 74% starch and 11% fiber. Therefore, they contain mostly starch, and the name "principal starch" is the most apt term.

[14] Mintz SW (1985). Ibid, p. 10, Discussed in Chapter 1, Food, Sociality, and Sugar, especially pp. 9–13, also see references cited by Mintz, especially: Richards AI (1939). *Land, Labour and Diets in Northern Rhodesia,* pp. 46–49. London: Oxford University Press; Rozin E, Rozin P(1981). Culinary themes and variations. *Natural History* 90: 6–14.

with water and cooked. In some cases a flour was made and prepared as a bread, cake, or tortilla. Potatoes and rice could be boiled and eaten directly.

History of Principal Starches

Wheat was domesticated in the Fertile Crescent around 9000–8000 BC. However, the knowledge of how to process plants that were good sources of principal starches (containing both complex carbohydrates—starch and fiber) was known much earlier than this. In the Fertile Crescent, the first evidence of the processing of wild grain was dated to as early as 19000 BC, when basalt bowls and pestles (basically heavy crude rocks that fit together) were found at the archeological sites of ancient camps that bordered on the Sea of Galilee. Later, mortar and pestles (more highly designed and easier to manipulate grinding rocks), dating to 15000 BC, were discovered by archeologists in caves at the site known as Geometric Kebaran in the Southern Levant.[15]

Even today, farmers in the high Andes Mountains of Peru use smooth stone tables and a "big half-moon–shaped stone" (see diagram in the chapter on Fiber) to hand grind quinua (also spelled quinoa), a grain that "grows well above timberline, tolerating frost and drought and turning every color of autumn leaves as it ripens."[16]

In some cases, principal starches needed to be processed in order to remove toxins. Manitoc (cassava) is a plant that contains a starchy tuber that contains poisonous cyanogenic glycosides. In order to make it safe to eat, the tuber needs to be finely grated and allowed to sit in its own juices so that enzymes can degrade the glycosides. The juices are squeezed out and the prepared flour can then be baked or fried. Although containing this poison, processed manitoc is the principal starch for 800 million people today, mainly in South America and Africa.[17]

The rough processing of complex carbohydrates from plants such as grains, tubers, and collected seed pods produced principal starch foods that still contained a significant amount of plant connective materials or cell walls from the plants. Humans consumed roughly ground grains as part of coarse breads or as a filler in porridge.

---

[15] Bellwood P (2005). *First Farmers: The Origins of Agricultural Societies.* Malden, MA: Blackwell Publishing, p. 51.

[16] McIntyre L (1975). *The Incredible Incas and Their Timeless Land.* Washington, DC: The National Geographic Society, quotes from pages 50 and 48.

[17] Silvertown J (2017). *Dinner with Darwin: Food, Drink, and Evolution.* Chicago: University of Chicago, p. 109.

Since humans who practiced agriculture thrived on crops that largely provided principal starches, it is reasonable to suggest that human metabolism evolved to become finely tuned to their efficient digestion, storage, and utilization of the calories. This included the ability of the human intestine to handle the high amounts of fiber that came along with a principal starch.[18]

Therefore, we must conclude that humans were sophisticated consumers and manipulators of principal starches for at least 10,000 years before the introduction of new sources of calories, such as sugar (which was added to the diet of most people in England for the very first time starting in the mid-1700s when sugar was commonly added to tea and coffee), and much later, when vegetable oils were introduced (which were produced in bulk for the very first time in the late 1800s after the introduction of modern milling equipment allowed the efficient extraction of plant oils—mainly from seeds).

There are three important events that greatly influenced the transition to more modern American diets. First, at around 700 BC, there is the appearance of sugarcane in India. Actually, sugarcane originated in New Guinea, which was one of the other areas that independently developed sophisticated agriculture.[19] Second, is 1776, when the American colonies revolted from England. This year is important for another reason—James Watt demonstrated his steam engine in England in 1776, thus spurring the industrial revolution. And third, mechanical roller milling technology was brought to America in the 1870s and, **it** was so much more efficient than stone grinding, that by 1880 almost all of the large grain mills on the Mississippi River at Minneapolis used roller milling to produce flour.

Invention of Mechanical Steel Roller Milling for Grain

The mechanical roller milling machine was invented in Hungary in the 1860s and later improved in several countries in Europe.[20] The new method, the "Hungarian method," included finely spaced steel rollers, that could be adjusted to grind wheat into different flour grades. The steel rollers lasted longer than the grinding stones and could be adjusted to produce the desired product. Also, they produced less heat than the large grinding stones, and therefore the flour was not damaged or discolored as much. The acceptance of white flour for making bread and baking was a critical change in the diets of Americans.

[18] Hardy K, Brand-Miller J, Brown KD, Thomas MG, Copeland L (2015). The importance of dietary carbohydrate in human evolution. *Q Rev Biol* 90(3): 251–268. https://www.ncbi.nlm.nih.gov/pubmed/26591850

[19] Diamond J. See books, including: Diamond J (1997). *Guns, Germs, and Steel: The Fates of Human Societies.* New York: W. W. Norton; and Diamond J (2011). *Collapse: How Societies Choose to Fail or Succeed.* (Revised Edition). New York: Penguin Books.

[20] Perren R (1990). Structural change and market growth in the food industry: flour milling in Britain, Europe, and America, 1850–1914. *Economic History Rev* 43(3): 420–443.

Previously I discussed the concept of a principal starch and how this also contained fiber! Next is a rough figure of a half kernel of grain. In the central area is the endosperm, or starch, which is stored energy for the new plant. This large portion of the kernel contains special cells that become packed with starch granules. On the outside is the protective covering called the bran, which is an excellent source of fiber. Right underneath the outer bran are cells that are enriched in the proteins that make up gluten. On the left middle is the germ, which will become the new plant. This is an excellent source of vitamins and minerals. And the straggly material on the right is plant structural material caught with the grain. The amount of plant material attached to the kernel is dependent upon the method of harvesting and pre-cleaning.

Half a Kernel of Grain

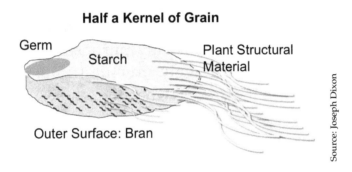

The next figure compares the hand milling of grain using a granite rock table and a "big half-moon–shaped stone" used as a pestle (left),[21] and a modern mechanical, motor-driven roller milling device (right).

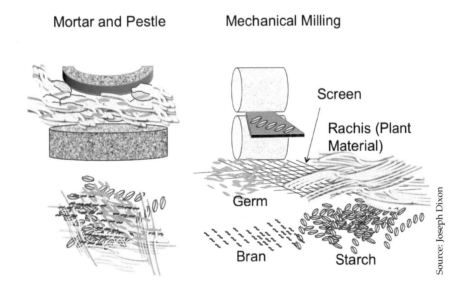

---

[21] McIntyre L (1975). *The Incredible Incas and Their Timeless Land.* Washington, DC: The National Geographic Society, p. 50.

In the first method (left side), the rough (or whole) grain is ground using this early mortar and pestle, and once ground, it is swept into a bowl and another batch is started on. It was difficult to separate the parts of the whole kernel (see all portions mixed together in the figure), so the early cook took the smoother material that gathered at the bottom of the bowl and used it as flour, and the top rougher material was used as thickener in a stew or porridge. In this way all of the rough grain could be used as food—usually that same day or in the next couple of days at the latest.

With mechanical roller milling machine (right side), the whole grain could be more finely milled and the different portions of the grain could be collected individually using screening. This allowed a more refined flour to be produced that could be stored longer before becoming rancid. The glutinous particles were collected and reground and added back to the flour. The germ (enriched in vitamins and minerals) could be collected and stored and sold separately. The bran could be collected and used for many purposes including nonfood uses such as bedding or fine pulp. The straggly structural material could also be used for pulp or discarded early in the process when the whole grain was mechanically pre-cleaned.

The problem with this last process is that for 10,000 years, humans had become adapted to eating a principal starch that had been hand ground, and thus, it contained a very–high-fiber content as well as the germ portion of the grain. When modern milling was established in most western nations, the highly efficient method of processing a large tonnage of grain quickly and more uniformly became part of the fabric of modern agriculture. The losses of the important components (germ and bran) from the whole grain were not even considered important at the time. But, in fact, these losses were extremely important and changed the entire framework of nutrition. What we have been eating for the past 100 years or so is a radical departure from what humans ate during the entire previous 10,000 years of agriculture.

Below is a table (derived from Table 2.1 of William Atwell's book)[22] that shows the content of selected nutrients in whole wheat grain, white flour made by milling wheat using modern roller milling, and the same white flour after it has been enriched with certain nutrients. The down facing red arrows show the loss of nutrients after white flour is produced. The nutrients with the red Es are some of the nutrients that are enriched by law.

---

[22] Atwell W, Finnie S (2016). *Wheat Flour,* Second Edition, Elsevier Science & Technology, Chapter 2, p. 26.

Loss of Nutrients in Wheat During the Modern Milling Process

Nutritional Content of Whole-Grain, Unenriched White Flour, and Enriched White Flour[a]

Nutrient	Whole-Grain	White Flour (Unenriched)	White Flour (Enriched)
Protein (g/100 g)	12.73	11.54	11.54
Lipid (g/100 g)	2.41	1.6	1.6
Carbohydrate (g/100 g)	69.34	69.88	69.88
Fiber (g/100 g)	10.31	2.31	2.31
Calcium (mg/100 g)	32.76	14.45	14.45
Iron (mg/100 g)	3.47	0.87	4.25 E
Magnesium (mg/100 g)	132	24.09	24.09
Potassium (mg/100 g)	349.74	96.35	96.35
Sodium (mg/100 g)	1.93	1.93	1.93
Thiamin (mg/100 g)	0.48	0.08	0.78 E
Niacin (mg/100 g)	4.78	0.96	7.28 E
Vitamin A (mg/100 g)	8.67	1.93	1.93
Vitamin K (mg/100 g)	1.83	0.29	0.29

[a] Data from USDA Food National Nutrient Database.

This table shows only a selection of nutrients. ↓ indicates nutrient was lost with milling. E indicates the nutrient was added back (Enriched) to the flour.

Source: Joseph Dixon

The nutrients that are listed in the second column of numbers show how poor nutritionally white flour is compared to whole grain that is described in the first column. The overall conclusion is that for over 100 years, products made from mechanically milled white flour have been providing a poor spectrum of nutrients, especially a very much lower fiber content, to the American diet. In my mind this is one of the most important factors that set up the Obesity Explosion that was to come.

Factors that Led up to the Obesity Explosion

The Obesity Explosion is the result of an accumulation of many changes in our foods and how they were processed, advertised, and sold. In the period 1870–1880, there was a veritable earthquake in food processing when the almost 20 large grain mills in the Minneapolis area converted to roller milling technology. The owners of the grain mills in Minneapolis only knew that mechanical roller milling increased the speed of the milling process and produced a product (white flour) that possessed a much longer shelf life. Also, the consumers loved this new kind of flour. Therefore, the owners could make more money and did not realize that bleached refined flour lost a large amount of the nutrients in the original grain. After all, the first vitamin was not discovered until around 1911. The decreased intakes in fiber and nutrients due to the use of refined flours was one of the first major changes in the food supply that caused negative effects on health and laid the foundation for the Obesity Explosion. But it was not the last.

The table at the end of the previous chapter clearly showed how white flour is much poorer nutritionally than wholegrain flours—even today. In this chapter we continue the journey on how food changed in the 80 to 100 years before the Obesity Explosion.

On the Timeline below I have placed many singular events over the past 150 years that are not usually considered in the current discussions of obesity, but which I think are important to the run up to the Obesity Explosion.

Factors Leading Up To The Obesity Explosion

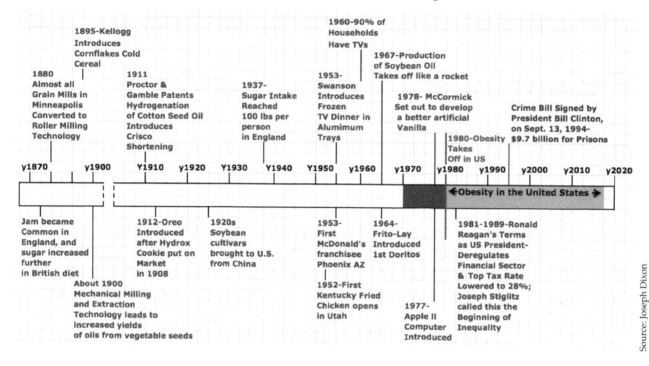

Source: Joseph Dixon

Before we enter this timeline, I just need to go back and highlight an earlier major change in our diet. It turns out that sugar is a rather late comer to our diet. The Romans did not have sugar. Sugar arrived in the port city of Venice from India just before 1000 AD. And only the very rich in Europe could afford sugar during the Middle Ages. Sometime between 1650 and 1750, sugar became an important part of the diets of most people in Great Britain, and this later flowed over to its American colonists. In England sugar was used in coffee and tea and in new foods such as jams and confections. I will discuss the possible role of sugar in the Obesity Explosion later in this book.

Looking at the timeline, it shows that by 1880 American grain mills had largely converted to the new roller mill technology imported from Hungry and Germany. The new technology produced flour more efficiently than stone grinding. But once it was observed that new technologies could be used to revolutionize grain milling, entrepreneurs searched for other ways to manipulate and sell farm products.

In 1895, Kellogg discovered that corn could be flattened and then roasted to produce a crispy and tasty flake that was delicious when combined with sugar and milk. Kellogg introduced a prepackaged Cornflakes cold cereal that immediately became popular. This led to the introduction of other kinds of cereal made from different refined grains. Eventually, a cereal industry was created that thrived on mechanical milling and adding sugar and other components (such as raisins) to cereals. There would be mass marketing of highly colored packages of sugar-containing cereals to children on another new technology, television.

In the early 1900s the new mechanical roller–grain-refining technology was adapted to the extraction of seeds to produce vegetable oils. This was a leap forward with tremendous consequences. Up until this time, seeds from many crops had been considered a useless byproduct. For example, after the harvest, the seeds from cotton had just been discarded for ages. But with the new mechanical technologies, the oil from cotton seeds could be extracted and recovered with good efficiency. The next question was, "What to do with the cottonseed oil?" From 1900–1910 Proctor & Gamble worked to perfect the hydrogenation (hardening) of vegetable oils, and in 1911, they released Crisco (short for Crystallized Cotton seed Oil) as a shortening that could be used in cooking (especially baking). Therefore, a very cheap, previously unused natural product, cottonseed oil, could be transformed into a valuable product that was used by Americans to bake pies and prepare other foods. Just as an aside, the legal battles over the patents awarded to Proctor & Gamble for the hydrogenation (hardening) of vegetable oils were some of the most ferocious litigation of the early 20th century. But the successful utilization of cottonseed oil for baking would start a revolution in the food industry. Vegetable oils would become powerful components of the food industry and the American diet. And the Calories that are present in vegetable oils would also have a great effect.

In 1912, the National Biscuit Company (Nabisco) introduced the Oreo cookie and made them in a bakery in the Chelsea neighborhood of Manhattan, New York. The Oreo followed the introduction of the Hydrox cookie that was first marketed in 1908 by Sunshine. The Oreo would go on to become the most popular cookie in America, with over 30 varieties of Oreo being introduced at different times. If you visit New York City, you can visit the Chelsea Market, which occupies a large building between Ninth and Tenth Avenues and 15th and 16th streets in Manhattan. This building was the site of the National Biscuit Company where the first Oreos were made, and as you walk through the market, you can read about the making of Oreo cookies.

In the 1920s and 1930s soybean cultivars were brought to the U.S. from China. The soybean plant is not native to North America, but it is found throughout Southeast Asia. Various cultivars of soybeans were brought to North America and agronomists chose and fostered varieties that would thrive in American soils. Farmers came to love growing soybeans because this crop also adds nitrogen back into soil (in a process called nitrogen fixation) in a safe and cost effective way. After a decade of learning how to grow soybeans, farmers began to produce soybeans in commercial quantities and in the 1940s soybean oil appeared on the market. Production of soybean oil increased greatly in the 1960s in order to fulfill the demand for cooking oils from the newly establish fast-food industry in the U.S. As I often say in my class, soybean oil and fast food are like a horse and carriage—"You can't have one without the other!"

In 1937, the intake of sugar in Great Britain reached 100 pounds/person/year. A major result of this was a whole generation of the English who grew up with poor teeth due to dental caries. The intake of sugar in the U.S. was less documented at this time, but was probably less than that observed in Great Britain.

After World War II, American industry was directed into automobile production and a direct result was that the American family hit the highways that were being built at the same time. In order to feed the American family on the road, two powerhouse franchise restaurant chains were established in the 1950s. After years of making fried chicken for local consumption in Kentucky, Colonel Sanders opened the first Kentucky Fried Chicken franchise restaurant in Utah in 1952. And just the next year, after years of experimentation in southern California, the first McDonald's franchise was opened in Phoenix AZ in 1953. Also in 1953, with a surplus of turkeys on their hands, Swanson foods introduced the frozen TV dinner in aluminum trays. This dinner was designed to be popped in the oven and then eaten in front of the Television set. On the timeline you can see that in 1960, 90% of homes contained a television set.

In 1964, Texas-based Frito-Lay introduced Doritos corn chips. At first they were a complete failure. Only after the chip was formulated to taste similar to a tasty taco did sales of Doritos take off in the U.S. In the mid-1960s, the production of soybean oil took off like a rocket—probably in order to supply the needs of the growing fast food and snack industries with cooking oil (see the coming commodities chapters). The success of Doritos corn chips led other companies to develop other varieties of baked snack chips and crackers. This influenced the intake of grain in the U.S.

In 1977, Apple computer introduced the Apple II computer designed and built by Steve Wozniak. This computer revolutionized the desktop computer because it was much easier to use and was adaptable for many useful purposes. In 1982, I wrote my Ph.D. the old fashioned way, using hand writing and then a type writer. At the very same time a lab mate of mine used an Apple IIe to write his Ph.D. thesis. I will always remember the advantage of using even a simple desktop computer to write a very complicated document.

All of the above events listed on the timeline had significant effects on American life and eating. In 1978, an event occurred that, after a fair delay, would greatly affect the nature of foods sold throughout our country. In 1978, the price of vanilla beans skyrocketed due to the destruction of plantations in Madagascar as a result of war. The spice and flavor company, McCormick, initiated the search for, and the development of, an artificial vanilla flavoring. In one of McCromick research laboratories, a gifted lab technician, Marianne Gillette, discovered an important compound in natural vanilla extract that is important to the taste and feel of real vanilla flavoring. Using modern chemical flavors, McCormick marketed in 1982 a successful synthetic vanilla flavoring. This led to the epiphany that any taste or flavoring could be reproduced using a mixture of the approximate 2,500 synthetic chemicals that were available to the food industry. This "idea" spawned the development of a whole new spectrum of flavors and foods. The discovery that such an important flavoring could be replaced by a mixture of chemicals could be considered the genie being let out of the flavor bottle. From then on, the American appetite would be fueled by foods developed by food wizards in the laboratories of the food industry. The discovery of artificial vanilla was the ignition of the fuse that exploded the Obesity bomb.

On or around 1980, the steady increase in the body weight of Americans began, leading to the Obesity Explosion described throughout this book. Everything mentioned so far, and many factors that I have not yet mentioned, went into the dynamite that fueled the explosion. The discovery by McCormick lit the fuse, and the American food industry learned that it could use chemistry to expand our brains with flavors and delicious odors of every type.

Role of Culture and Inequality in Sustaining What the Obesity Explosion Over the Next 40 Years

It the Obesity Explosion started in 1980, it was the period immediately afterwards that allowed it to fester and accelerate. Many large cultural changes erupted in the American way of living.

In 1981, President Ronald Reagan began his first term as President of the United States. Dr. Joseph Stiglitz, Nobel winning economist, called President Reagan's deregulation of the financial sector, and the lowering of the top tax rate to 28%, as the "Beginning of Inequality." A later chapter in this book will describe how Income Inequality continues the cycle of the Obesity Explosion.

On November 9, 1989, the Berlin Wall fell and with it the beginning of the end of communism in Eastern Europe. It appeared that American Power would become supreme and the United States might benefit from not having a dangerous adversary in the Soviet Union. The United States could now spend its wealth on the reconstruction of the country's infrastructure that has been allowed to fall into disarray during the arms race. But then something happened that put that noble idea on a different track. On September 13, 1994, President Bill Clinton signed the Violent Crime Control and Law Enforcement Act of 1994. This bill called for

$9.7 billion in funding for the building of new prisons. The increased severity of sentencing laws increased the incarceration rates in the U.S. to the highest rate in the Western world. The more men in prison, the more single parent households were created in America. This law supplemented harsher sentencing laws that were enacted in the earlier 1970s in response to President Nixon's War on Crime. Because federal funds were not earmarked for prisoner maintenance, individual states needed to shift money from other priorities such as education to take care of prisoners. Therefore, funds that had been used to support education and public colleges were withdrawn to pay for the incarceration of prisoners, a large majority of whom were men of color. In an ironic and sad reality, the cost of keeping one prisoner in prison per year amounted to about twice the cost of sending a student to college for a year.

Here are some of the noticeable changes that occurred after the above timeline was completed:

1. Economics changed so that both caregivers had to work and less healthy dinners were made in the home.
2. Children did not learn to cook from their mother or father.
3. Fast-food restaurants proliferated so that they are almost everywhere.
4. Two powerful digital systems were introduced into the home—the television and the computer.
5. Supermarkets became extraordinary large and started to sell convenience foods of every kind.
6. Food companies learned how to make their products super palatable.
7. Food companies expanded their product lines so that there were foods for every taste.
8. Manufacturers moved out of the US so that there were less blue-collar jobs that needed significant energy expenditure.
9. Computers became ubiquitous in every work situation.
10. Automobiles proliferated such that some families have three to four cars.
11. Work-saving devices of every kind were developed.
12. Air conditioning made it much more comfortable to sit inside in the summer.

The years since 1994 have included an intensification of all the factors that had come before. Now that we recognize the many different aspects of the era of obesity, we can make some informed guesses about how and why the increase in per capita food Calories occurred throughout the U.S.

The food supply did in fact change drastically during this whole time period and this definitely had an effect on food intake and Calorie intake. Models indicate that daily Calorie intake increased to as high as 280 calories per day (kcal) in Americans who achieved the higher levels of obesity seen today (2020). And smaller increases in daily kilocalorie intake, maybe as little as 100 kcal/day can be responsible for smaller increases in weight that led people to enter the overweight category or to just over the obesity mark as denoted by a BMI of 30 or slightly above. What these observations say is that what appears to be a relatively small increase in the daily intake of approximately 100 to 300 kcal/day could explain the current Obesity Explosion. This is one reason it fell under the radar. Little by little the jolts to weight maintenance added up.

Changes in the Sources of Carbohydrates and Protein Over the Past 150 Years

Did any one food cause the Obesity Explosion? Can we track down a commodity that increased greatly in the 1900s such that Americans were eating more Calories per day? Was it carbohydrate, or more specifically, sugar that caused the large increase in average weight?

The introduction of sugar into extended English society in the mid-1700s (spurred on by the popularity of the new beverages, coffee and tea) caused an earthquake in English diets. Similarly, the diets of Americans were greatly altered in the past 100 years or so by changes in the processing of grains. The introduction of mechanical roller technology into the U.S. in the 1880s led to the wide spread use of processed, refined grain products (including breakfast cereals). And later on, advances in carbohydrate chemistry led to the consumption of enzyme-produced sweeteners derived from corn starch. From then on, American diets and physiques slowly changed and would never be the same.

Changes in Calorie Intake during the Obesity Explosion

Since Calories count, let's first look at how Calorie intake changed during the 40 years or so when the Obesity Explosion occurred. As most nutritionists know, determining how many Calories a person eats on a daily basis is extremely difficult. Food recall and food diary methods have been proven to be highly unreliable. On a country basis, there are several different ways to estimate daily Calorie intake for the population. Just like the census, certain allowances need to be interjected to provide a corrected, but probably a more accurate value. In the figure below, Calorie intake is derived from the U.S. Department of Agriculture (USDA) food availability data[1] that were corrected for spoilage, and it shows an increase in intake of about 550 kcal/person/day between 1970 and 2004. However, almost all experts have concluded that a 550-kcal increase per day per person is highly improbable. At this level of intake, most of us would be of a very large size. And getting accurate figures for how much food goes unused in the U.S. is very difficult, if not impossible. Also, availability data tends to overestimate intake, whereas survey data tends to underestimate intake (by 30% in some studies). The accurate intake of Calories is probably somewhere in between. So another approach was needed to determine how much Calorie intake increased per person per day during the Obesity Explosion.

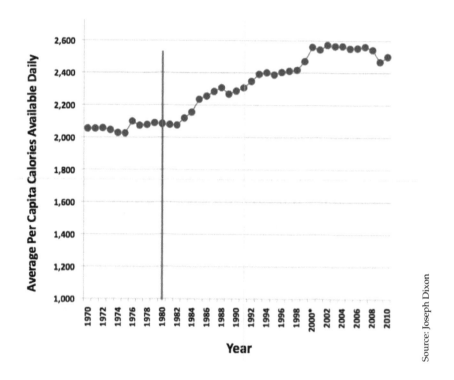

Source: Joseph Dixon

Since overall food availability data did not provide accurate data on Calorie intake changes during the past 40 years, Dr. Kevin Hall's research group at the Laboratory of Biological Modeling, National Institute of Diabetes and Digestive and Kidney Diseases, took a different approach. Dr. Hall's group calculated, using the increase in average body weights of adults over the past 30 years from National

---

[1] Calculated by ERS/USDA based on data from various sources (see https://www.ers.usda.gov/data-products/food-availability-per-capita-data-system/loss-adjusted-food-availability-documentation/). Data last updated June 1, 2019. Note: Per capita Total Calorie Availability for after 2010 was not available in the USDA database when last checked in May 2020. The red vertical line denotes the Obesity Explosion in 1980.

Health and Nutrition Examination Survey (NHANES) survey data, that per capita kilocalorie intake increased from a baseline value in 1973 by the amounts shown in the figure below.[2,3] Throughout this book, the year 1980 has been designated as when the Obesity Explosion occurred, and Dr. Hall's research group calculated that Americans consumed about 40 kcal extra per person per day for the year 1980. But as the Obesity Explosion continued, the graph shows that the amount of extra Calories consumed per day increased in a linear fashion. Dr. Hall's calculation of the extra Calories consumed as the Obesity Explosion reached the year 2010 amounted to about 280 kcal/person/day. This value fits experimentally gathered data from several other studies, and is much more reasonable, than the calculations carried out using the countrywide commodity availability data. Because the data

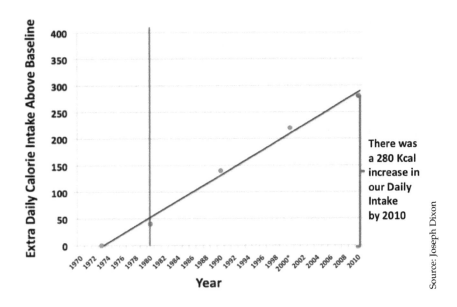

Source: Joseph Dixon

The values (blue circles) are the calculated energy intake changes that would explain the weight gain observed in the U.S. population over this period of time. See Footnote for Hall KD, Guo J, Dore M, Chow CC. (2009). From the Methods Section: "…the average initial energy intake was I0 (Initial energy intake) = 2,100 kcal/day calculated using the energy requirement equations of the Institute of Medicine of the National Academies [33] for a sedentary population corresponding to the average demographics of the initial adult NHANES population." The Initial energy intake was set to zero for the year 1973 for graphical purposes. Any values above zero on the graph are the amount required to support the increase in weight during the Obesity Explosion.

[2] Hall KD, Guo J, Dore M, Chow CC (2009). The progressive increase of food waste in America and its environmental impact. *PLoS One* 4:e7940. https://www.ncbi.nlm.nih.gov/pubmed/19946359

[3] Kevin DHl (2018). Did the food environment cause the obesity epidemic? *Obesity* 26, 11–13. https://www.ncbi.nlm.nih.gov/pubmed/29265772

calculated by Dr. Hall's group appears more reasonable and can be more strongly supported, I will use 280 kcal/person/day throughout the rest of this book when I try to assign operational blame on a particular lifestyle or food pattern for the Obesity Explosion.

Why the concept that Calorie Consumption Increased by an Average Value of 280 kcal/person/day by 2010 is the Most Important Fact in this Book

First, the data presented in the graph indicates that the increase in Calorie consumption started slowly, therefore making it difficult to see a difference around 1980. Second, the increase in Calorie consumption was sustained such that as years went by, the average person in the U.S. consumed more and more Calories per day. Third, even by 2010, 30 years into the Obesity Explosion, the increase in Calorie consumption (280 cal/person/day) was not all that great on a relative scale basis. Realistically, it would be difficult to track a 280-cal difference in the intakes of individuals and groups participating in nutrition studies, and it would be extremely difficult to track differences free living populations across the U.S.

The rest of this chapter attempts to use data from the USDA in order to monitor which commodities increased during the Obesity Explosion, and which decreased during the same period of time. The assumption here is that tracking many different commodities followed by the economists of the USDA will provide insights into what foods increased during the Obesity Explosion, and therefore, may allow us to synthesize hypotheses concerning what foods were involved in the Obesity Explosion.

Changes in Carbohydrate Consumption during the 1900s and Early 2000s

As stated previously, in 1937 the intake of sugar in Great Britain averaged about 100 lb/person/year—much higher than it ever reached in the U.S. The data for the intake of sugar and other caloric sweeteners in the U.S. became more reliable after national surveys were instituted. In 1970, the intake of all sweeteners in the U.S. was about 67 lb/person/year, and it edged up until the year 2000, when it reached its peak at about 84 lb/person/year. Then intake went back down.

The full data for the intake of sweeteners (Calories per person per day) in the U.S., based upon USDA commodity information,[4] is shown in the next figure.

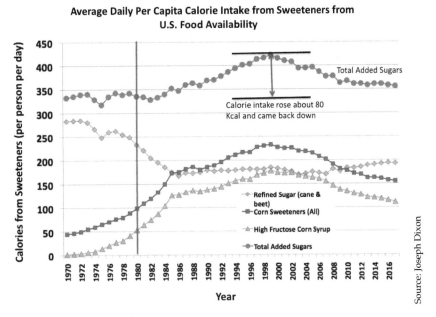

Source: Calculated by ERS/USDA based on data from various sources (see https://www.ers.usda.gov/data-products/food-availability-per-capita-data-system/loss-adjusted-food-availability-documentation/). Data last updated June 1, 2019. For information contact Linda Kantor at linda.kantor@ers.usda.gov or Jeanine Bentley at jbentley@ers.usda.gov for more information.

I have also included a breakdown of the contributions that refined sugar from sugar cane and beets, and sweeteners obtained from processing corn, played in Calorie intake. Intake of total added sweeteners increased by about 70 to 80 Calories from 1970 to 2000, but then, consumption started to fall and, by the year 2010, intake of sweeteners had almost reached the value previously observed in 1970. What is shocking, and this has been discussed in many articles in the obesity field, is the increase in the contributions of corn sweeteners, especially High-Fructose Corn Syrup (HFCS), to the total added sweeteners consumed per day by Americans.

However, the overall impression given by this figure is that the increase in daily Calories from all added sweeteners (red double arrow) was moderate between years 1970 and 2000 (only about 80 kcal/day at most), and then started to decline thereafter.

---

[4] Economic Research Service, U.S. Department of Agriculture (ERS/USDA). http://www.ers.usda.gov/data-products/food-availability-%28per-capita%29-data-system/.aspx

When we compare, on a daily basis, the above Sweetener kilocalorie intake data with total kilocalorie consumption data presented previously for the target year of 2000, total Calorie intake increased by 220 kcal, whereas the maximal increase in total sweeteners increased by about 80 kcal, which was about 38% of the total kilocalorie increase. So you could say that intake of sweeteners may have contributed to the Obesity Explosion. But at other times during the period, especially closer to 1980, the increase in sweetener consumption did not even approach that of the increase in the daily total kilocalorie intake.

Putting the two types of observations together over the whole period, it is apparent that the increase in total sweetener consumption cannot explain a large part of the Obesity Explosion. The story is much more complicated than blaming all of obesity on sugar consumption, as some "Internet Nutrition Experts" have proposed.

If the increase in Calories due to sweeteners (about 80 kcal/day) cannot explain the increase in total Calories per day measured during the Obesity Explosion, what foods or commodities were increased during the past 50 years? The changes in the major food commodity groups according to the USDA are shown in the next two graphs.[5]

A) Food Groups that decreased:

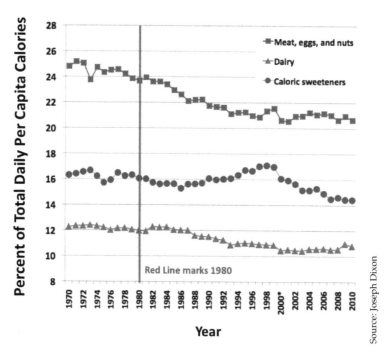

[5] Source: Calculated by ERS/USDA based on data from various sources (see https://www.ers.usda.gov/data-products/food-availability-per-capita-data-system/loss-adjusted-food-availability-documentation/). Data last updated June 1, 2019. Due to the termination of select Current Industrial Reports (CIR) by the Census Bureau, data on some added fats and oils could not be updated beyond 2010 in the Food Availability Data System. This means that certain summary estimates—such as per capita daily amounts of calories and food pattern equivalents (or servings)—cannot be calculated beyond 2010 for the added fats & oils group. Additionally, the summary estimates or totals across all food groups cannot be calculated beyond 2010. The Red vertical line at 1980 denotes the Obesity Explosion.

B) Food Groups that increased:

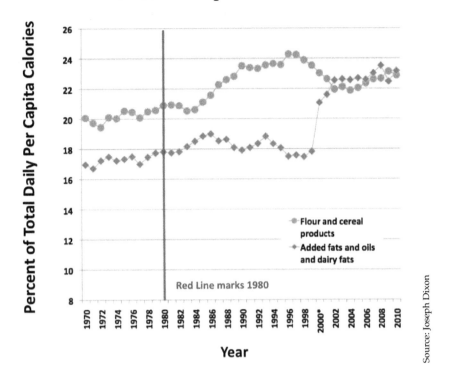

Source: Joseph Dixon

The data were plotted on two graphs for clarity. Not shown on either graph are the contributions from Fruit and Vegetables. These two commodities were below 8% of total daily Calories and their intake were very consistent throughout the entire period. When the major food groups are graphed during the rise in obesity, three groups (Panel A) actually went down as percent of total daily Calories: Meat, eggs, and nuts; Dairy; and caloric sweeteners. Although in the previous graph Caloric sweeteners remained fairly consistent as Calories per person per day, because total Calorie consumption increased, the actual Percent of total daily Calories from sweeteners decreased. Two food groups in particular showed a substantial increase during this period. Panel B: Flour and cereal products (yellow circles) increased steadily from 1972 through 1995. At around 1996, this group started to slightly decline as fats increased stunningly. And Added fats, oils, and dairy fats, increased during the rise in obesity (light blue diamonds), but in a more complicated way. It increased steadily and slowly from 1970 through 1986, then leveled off in a haphazard way until the mid-1990s, when it shot up again, possibly due to a different level of reporting (see asterisk and footnote), and possibly as a counter reaction to the earlier fat phobia movement of the 1980s to 1990s.[6] In fact, the Added fats, oils, and dairy

---

[6] Was there fat phobia in the 1990s? I remember very clearly that college students in my nutrition classes in the 1990s projected a strong fear of dietary fat such that the average intake of total Calories from fat was about 25% for this group when I graded their dietary assignments over a ten year period. However, as much of the increase in fat intake was due to fast food (due to shortening, soy oil, and chicken), then if the students refrained from fast food during the assignment, their intakes of fat would have been artificially low.

fats group increased dramatically from 1998 to 2002. In this short time period, daily Calories due to added fats increased from 18% to about 23% of total daily Calorie intake. When graphed as Per Capita Calorie Intake, the increase in Calorie intake due to added fats, oils, and dairy fat amounted to about 300 cal between 1970 and 2010. A more detailed look at fat consumption will be addressed in the next chapter.

For now, let's look at the increases in flour, cereal, and grains. Below is a graph of total grain availability and the individual grains that make up total grain intake in the U.S.

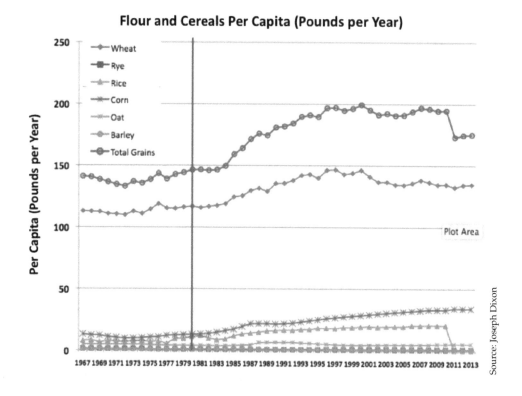

Total grain availability per capita (red circles) increased a resounding 50 lb/person/year from 1967 to 2013. Looking at individual grains, one can see that wheat and corn increased the most, followed by rice. The next graph shows wheat and corn flour availability on the same graph as potato availability. This time the data is presented as Daily Per Capita Calories for each.

Average Daily Per Capita Calories of Wheat, Corn, and Potatoes

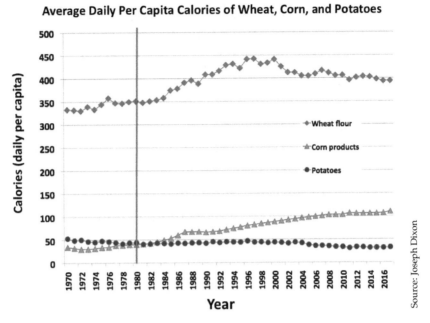

Source: Joseph Dixon

The values are average daily per capita calories from the U.S. food availability, adjusted for spoilage and other waste. Wheat included white, whole, and Durum flours. Corn includes flour, meal, hominy, grits, and cornstarch. Potatoes includes fresh and dehydrated. Calculated by ERS/USDA based on data from various sources (see https://www.ers.usda.gov/data-products/food-availability-per-capita-data-system/loss-adjusted-food-availability-documentation/). Data last updated June 1, 2019. Red Vertical Bar at 1980 denotes the Obesity Explosion.

Wheat flour availability increased about 25% during the time period and corn availability increased by about 100%! Because wheat started out as supplying more Calories, it actually supplied the greater increase in Calories per person per year. The mass increase in corn availability was about 12.5 lb/person/year. The increase in Calories due to corn products (and most likely intake) is stunning. Around 1980 corn was steadily increasing, and then in 1984, the availability of corn products really took off. In 1989, the yearly increases in corn flour availability resumed to the previous rate seen around 1980. The success of corn chips as a snack food can be gauged by Frito-Lay's support of college football's Fiesta Bowl in Arizona from 1996 through 2014. According to Wikipedia[7] Frito-Lay developed Tostitos using the same cooking method used in Mexico, giving them an authentic taste. The brand was launched in 1980 and was hugely successful. The Bowl's name during this time was called the Tostitos Fiesta Bowl.

---

[7] Wikipedia, the free encyclopedia. Accessed on January 11, 2018. https://en.wikipedia.org/wiki/Tostitos

In contrast to corn products, it was very surprising to find that the potato Calories did not change that much over this period. The next graph shows the retail disappearance of fresh potatoes in pounds per capita per year. In fact, starting around 2004, there was a fair decrease in potato usage in the country. This is surprising because of the apparent ubiquitous presence of potato chips in supermarkets and French fries in fast-food restaurants. However, it is true that snack food products made from corn and wheat may have cut into the consumption of potato chips on a per capita basis. Also, this decrease may have been the result of a decrease in potato consumption in the home in the form of mashed potatoes, boiled potatoes, or baked potatoes (three of my favorites!). When presented as pounds of potatoes, usage also shows a drop beginning around 2004.

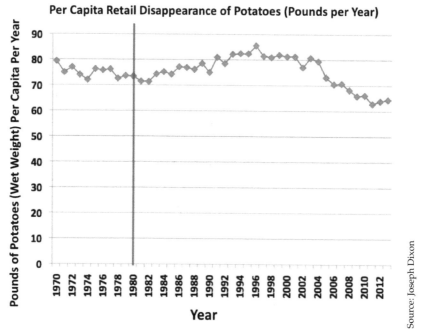

Source: Calculated by ERS/USDA based on data from various sources (see http://www.ers.usda.gov/data-products/food-availability-(per-capita)-data-system/food-availability-documentation.aspx). Data last updated February 1, 2015.

What is remarkable about the results presented in the above graphs is that while the "Internet nutrition experts" were screaming about the dangers of toxic sugar intake, major contributions to increased total calorie intake were coming from increased consumption of foods derived from highly processed grains! A majority of the increases in wheat and corn flour were due to the consumption of highly refined flours that have low-fiber content. Such products are mostly used in commercial bread baking and in the snack food industry.

Protein Availability throughout the 1900s and Protein Intake Based upon USDA Survey

Protein intake only provides a small percentage of a person's total energy intake per day—somewhere around 14% to 16% of total Calories per day. The consensus of most nutritionists is that the intake of protein is not a problem in the United States. We must remember that plants contain protein, and if there is increased consumption of grains, there must also be increased intake of protein. This is only common sense.

The protein available for consumption remained fairly level up until around 1976 when it shot up (see next graph). The values for the actual measured protein intake for males (denoted by the green triangle) and females (denoted by the green oval) are from data from several very large USDA survey studies.[8]

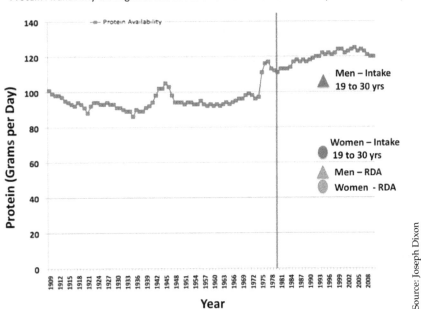

Protein Availability throughout the 1900s and Protein Intake Based upon USDA Survey

You can see that men (19 to 30 years old) consumed an average of 104 g of protein per day in 1994–1996, and women consumed 65 g of protein per day. Availability data tends to overestimate intake and survey data tends to underestimate intake (by 30% in some studies). The accurate intake of protein is probably somewhere in between.

[8] From U.S. food supply—Nutrients and other food components, per capita per day. Source: Calculated by USDA/Center for Nutrition Policy and Promotion. Data last updated February 1, 2015. Green triangle, Protein Intake (grams per day) in Men; Green oval, Protein Intake (grams per day) in women. Intake data from the USDA Continuing Survey of Food Intakes by Individuals 1994–96, 1998. Orange triangle, Protein RDA (grams per day) for Men, 19–30 years old; Orange oval, Protein RDA (grams per day) for Women, 19–30 years old. RDAs from Food and Nutrition Board (2005). Dietary Reference Intakes. Washington, DC: National Academies Press, see page 632. The red vertical line denotes 1980, the year where the Obesity Explosion appears to have taken off. Data were retrieved on December 16, 2016.

The graph indicates that the amount of protein available in the U.S. is much greater than either actual dietary intake or the Recommended Dietary Allowance (RDA - a reference value) for protein. Men consume a much higher amount of protein compared to the male RDA. Women also eat more than their RDA. Also note that since there is 4 kcal/g of protein, the increase in available Calories from protein over a long period of time, 1909–2010, amounts to about a total of 80 Calories.

What About the Intakes of Specific Protein-Rich Foods during the Obesity Explosion?

The following graph displays the intake of the major protein rich foods: Meat, Fish, Eggs, and Nuts. Quite interesting, the only food source that increased during the Obesity Explosion was poultry, which was offset by a decline in the consumption of Red Meats, which in this chart includes beef, pork, and lamb. The intake of nuts increased slightly; however, the intake of fish and shellfish remained extremely low. On the whole, total Calories from these sources of protein-rich foods, except for poultry, barely increased during the Obesity Explosion.

Meats, Eggs, and Nuts: Average Daily Per Capita Calories

Source: Joseph Dixon

Source: Calculated by ERS/USDA based on data from various sources (see https://www.ers.usda.gov/data-products/food-availability-per-capita-data-system/loss-adjusted-food-availability-documentation/). Data last updated June 1, 2019. The loss factors presented here are preliminary estimates and are intended to serve as a starting point for additional research and discussion. We welcome suggestions to expand on and improve our loss estimates. Red line denotes the Obesity Explosion.

Regarding the above graph, note that earlier I presented data that the percent Calories from total Meat, Eggs, and Nuts decreased during the Obesity Explosion. The earlier data decreased because total Calorie intake from all foods increased in the population during the same time, so the above results agree and make perfect sense. As you can see, Calories from Meat, Eggs, and Nuts did not increase, and therefore, are not part of the reasons for the Obesity Explosion.

The Calorie intake and commodity statistics presented in this chapter reveal several major changes in Calorie consumption and the use of common food products. The changes that strikingly stand out are:

1. Since 1973, the per capita daily intake of Calories increased such that by the year 2010, Americans were consuming about 280 more Calories per day per person than they did in 1973. This is the average Calorie increase calculated by the model. The calculated Calorie intake was averaged across the entire population, and it includes people who did not increase their calorie intake and people who increased their intake much more than 280 kcal/day. So it takes in the spectrum of responses.

2. Through most of the early part of the century there was a gradual decrease in the use of grains (mostly whole) with a late but modest upswing in the 1970–2000 period. The changes probably are a result of a decrease in the consumption of whole grains early, with a late upswing in the intake of highly milled grains later in the century.

3. There was also a gradual increase in the consumption of chicken starting in the period after World War II. Consumption of chicken increased throughout the rest of the century. This change was probably the result of increases in availability of chicken as large chicken farms were established at this time. The feeding practices of these large farms led to chickens that contained greater fat per chicken.

4. Interestingly, the per capita consumption of sugars stayed fairly consistent in the U.S. over the entire 1950–2000 period. This does not completely exonerate sugar as a causative factor of the Obesity Explosion. As will be discussed, the combination of sugar, sweeteners, fat, salt, and artificial and natural flavors were responsible for the production of super palatable foods and desserts.

When you go back to the beginning, it is an undeniable fact that humans have to consume more food per day in order for them to eat more Calories per day. This is not a chicken or the egg question. The results in this chapter show that is exactly what happened. But what is interesting is that the foods that increased in our diets are different than what is generally perceived.

The next chapter will discuss the intake of fats and oils in greater detail.

Changes in the Sources of Fat in Our Diet Over the Past 150 Years

Changes in Fat Consumption during the 1900s and Early 2000s

The Introduction of Vegetable Oils into the United States

In the timeline shown in Chapter 4, two momentous changes in the food science of fat occurred in the very early 1900s. In the late 1800s, in addition to other advances that occurred during the industrial revolution, modern milling equipment was developed and used to efficiently produce flour from grains. The basic milling machinery was continually improved, and it was eventually adapted to work with all different kinds of plant materials. It wasn't long before screw type processing equipment was developed and found to be very effective in processing hard materials such as plant seeds. It then became possible to extract vegetable oils from seeds in good yields. With more experience, food companies began to support the sale of a whole variety of vegetable oils and other products to replace the original cooking fats, such as lard, beef tallow, and palm oil that had been used up until that time. In one of the most important changes in the diet of Americans since the increased availability of sugar in the late 1600s to early 1700s, vegetable oils were introduced into the American diet. And soon afterwards, food companies experimented with the manipulations of vegetable oils in order to make them more suitable for use in the home. In 1911, Proctor & Gamble introduced Crisco, a beautiful glistening white, creamy semihard yet soft and smooth fat (called a shortening) that was perfect for use in baking. Not only was Crisco (short for Crystallized Cottonseed Oil) a useful and easy to use cooking fat, it had a long shelf life and looked very pure and ethereal. Because of its ease of use and the taste it imparted into breads and baked goods, American consumers fell in love with it.

The key to using cottonseed oil was the chemical process called hydrogenation, where hydrogen gas is pumped into liquid oil and, with the help of a catalyst, the fatty acids in the oil are made more saturated and the liquid oil is turned into a semihard substance that can be spread with a knife. Hydrogenation would also be used to make vegetable oils into margarine, a substitute for butter made from the cream of cow's milk. The results of these advances in food chemistry were the introduction of a whole line of new products that had never been available in the American diet. Americans no longer had to cook with greasy, smelly animal fats. They could buy a variety of cooking oils, shortenings like Crisco, and margarines of different consistencies. Only in the late 1900s would it become common knowledge (both among health professionals and the public) that the hydrogenation process produced unnatural fatty acids called trans fats. In fact, studies would show that trans-fatty acids were much more unhealthy than the usual saturated found in animal fats.

Blasbalg et al. reported on how the intake of omega-3 and omega-6 fatty acids changed in the American diet during the 1900s when the vast alterations in food fats occurred.[1] In order to study omega-3 and omega-6 intake, these researchers needed to give a panoramic look at what was being consumed in the U.S. during this time. In a series of figures, Blasbalg et al. charted how the use of fats and oils changed in the U.S. during the 20th century. I have chosen their Figure 1 (panels B and C) and Figure 2 to illustrate important changes in fat consumption. The first figure[2] shows how butter usage (blue line) decreased during the 1930s to the 1970s, and was replaced by increases in margarine (orange line) and shortening (red line) consumption. Lard (pig fat—also known as bacon fat) use (green line) also decreased greatly in the middle part of the 20th century. The steady increase in shortening use from the 1950s to 1990 probably reflects increased consumption of fast foods, where shortening was used in the frying of potatoes, chicken, and other foods, as well as increased usage in the home, where shortenings were used for frying and baking.

---

[1] Blasbalg TL, Hibbeln JR, Ramsden CE, Majchrzak SF, Rawlings RR (2011). Changes in consumption of omega-3 and omega-6 fatty acids in the United States during the 20th century. *Am J Clin Nutr* 93(5): 950–962. http://ajcn.nutrition.org/content/93/5/950.long

[2] This figure is from panel B of Figure 1 in Blasbalg *et al.* (2011). The original figure legend reads: Trends in the estimated per capita consumption of major food commodities (A), major fat commodities (B), and vegetable and seed oils (C) between 1909 and 1999. Kg/p/y, kilograms per person per year.

Changes in Table Fats Consumption

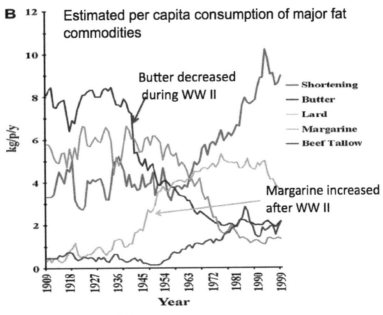

Am J Clin Nutr. 93(5): 950-962.

Whereas the previous figure showed hard fats, the second figure below (Panel C of Figure 1 from Blasbalg et al.) charts the use of vegetable oils (as liquids—not as part of shortening or margarine) through the 20th century. At the turn of the century, vegetable oil usage was very low in the U.S. diet. This of course reflects the difficulty in extracting seeds at this time. The use of vegetable oils increased slowly during the first half of the 1900s. Starting in the 1960s the use of soybean oil sky rocketed, increasing almost 10-fold. No other vegetable comes close to soybean oil in usage. In the late 1980s, canola oil, developed in Canada to replace palm oil imported from Southeast Asia, appeared on the U.S. market, and due to aggressive advertising, its use increased rapidly over the following 10 years. Note that the consumption of olive oil, which is high in monounsaturated fatty acids and one of the cornerstones of the Mediterranean diet, is not preferred in the U.S. and its consumption remained fairly low over the entire 20th century.

Changes in Vegetable Oil Consumption

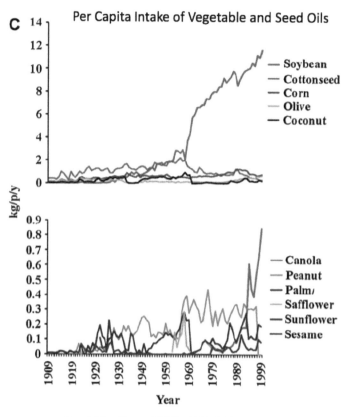

Am J Clin Nutr. 93(5): 950-962.

In the figure below (original Figure 2 in their paper), Blasbalg et al. compared all the major sources of Calories in the diet and depicted how their intakes varied over the 20th century. This figure is similar to what was presented earlier in previous chapter that focused on carbohydrate consumption. This graph shows the breakdown of foods slightly differently, and the period covered is much longer, almost the whole of the 20th century. The graph in the carbohydrate chapter showed that the per capita intake of added fats, oils, and dairy fats (added all together Calorie-wise) increased the most between 1970 and 2002. They were followed by flour and cereal products, which also increased. In the figure below from Blasbalg paper, the commodities are broken down more and the data over time period from 1909 to 1999 is more revealing. (1) The first general observation is that the foods consumed during the second half of the 1900s were widely different than the foods consumed during the first half of the 1900s. (2) The foods that increased from 1960 onward were shortening, soy oil, and poultry (which now often contains greater than 50% of Calories from fat in whole chickens, as well as reduced levels of omega-3 fatty acids compared to omega-6 fatty acids).[3]

---

[3] Wang Y, Lehane C, Ghebremeskel K, Crawford MA (2010). Modern organic and broiler chickens sold for human consumption provide more energy from fat than protein. *Public Health Nutrition* 13(3): 400–408. http://journals.cambridge.org/action/displayAbstract?fromPage=online&aid=7190300&fileId=S1368980009991157

(3) Intake of grains actually fell from 1909 to 1969 and then rebounded somewhat and increased from 1969 to 1999. The later increase in grains was probably due to the increased use of low-fiber processed flour in snack foods and cereals. (4) The increase in dairy during the first 50 years of the 1900s is interesting in terms of coronary heart disease (CHD). However, dairy decreased in the second half of the 1900s. Consumption of dairy and sugars were not the source of increased Calories from 1950 to 1999. (5) Beef and Pork intake had a roller coaster pattern over the whole century. Calories from vegetable products had a slight and steady decline over the entire century.

The data in the following figure is fairly definitive. The increase in consumption of Calories during the second half of the 20th century, the period when obesity increased in the U.S., was mostly due to increased consumption of fats and oils, increased consumption of chicken from 1960 to 1999, and increased consumption of grains (mostly wheat and corn) from 1970 to 1999.

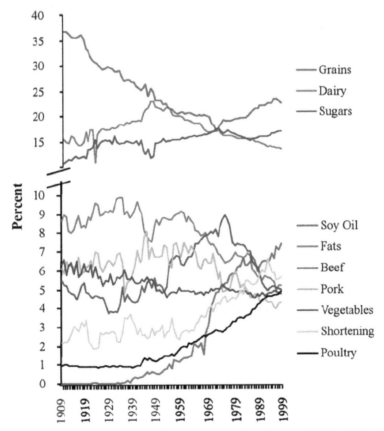

Year Am J Clin Nutr. 93(5): 950-962.

Major sources of calories between 1909 and 1999. Fats included shortening, butter, lard, margarine, and beef tallow. Soybean oil was considered separately from other oils because of its disproportionate contribution. Dairy included all milk, buttermilk, condensed milk, cream, sour cream, yogurt, cheese, and eggnog. Butter was not included in the dairy category to avoid double counting.

Although the 2011 article by Blasbalg, Hibbeln, Ramsden, Majchrzak, and Rawlings contained extensive consumption and availability data, these researchers were interested in determining the relative intake of omega-3 and omega-6 fatty acids. Their conclusions were:

By the end of the 1900s, the great increase in soybean oil consumption (showed above in several of the graphs) during the century increased linoleic acid (LA) (omega-6) from 2.79% to 7.21% of energy in fats, but increased α-linolenic acid (ALA) (omega-3) much less, from 0.39% to 0.72% of energy in fats. Therefore, the LA to ALA ratio in the food supply increased from 6.4 in 1909 to 10.0 in 1999. This translates to a much greater consumption in omega-6 fatty acids as the century progressed. Over the same time there were decreases in the consumption of arachidonic, eicosapentaenoic (EPA), and docosahexaenoic (DHA) fatty acids. The overall net effects of all these changes in the sources of fat during the 1900s was that LA (omega-6) intake increased and omega-3 EPA and DHA intakes decreased during the 20th century. The health effects of these changes are still being debated today. Some medical authorities believe that the long-term overall increase in the consumption of dietary omega-6 fatty acids has caused an increased general inflammatory state in our population.

Breakdown of the Added Fats and Oils Consumed at the Height of the Obesity Explosion

The data presented by Blasbalg et al. spanned almost the entire 20th century. We can make direct use of the USDA commodity tables in order to explore the new foodscape that was created by the Food Industry due to the massive transformation in the availability of new added edible fats and oils. This is shown in the following graph and pie charts. Not included in these charts are the fats that occur naturally within foods as they are eaten, such as fat in meat, vegetables, and nuts, and fat in drinkable milk products. This graph shows the use of "added fats," like those of salad and cooking oils, and shortening. The top line shows the Calories contributed by Total Added Fats. The total increase from 1970 to 2010 was about 250 total Calories—very close to the 280 Calories increase calculated by Dr. Hall's Group. The next line down shows that salad and cooking oils provided the major portion of edible added fats. Shortening increased after the year 1980 and increased throughout the remaining 1900s. But in 2004 shortening availability took a downturn.

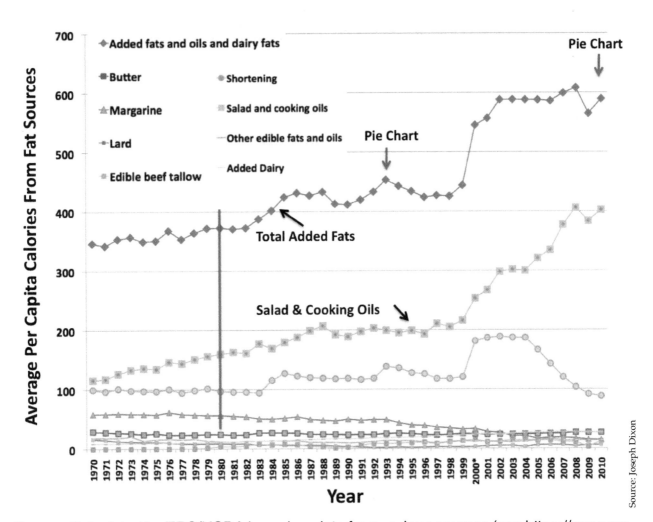

Source: Joseph Dixon

Source: Calculated by ERS/USDA based on data from various sources (see https://www.ers. usda.gov/data-products/food-availability-per-capita-data-system/loss-adjusted-food-availability-documentation/). Data last updated July 1, 2019. *In 2000, the number of firms reporting vegetable oil production to the Census Bureau increased, and this contributed to the spike in the data for salad and cooking oils, shortening, and aggregated numbers that use these estimates, such as total vegetable fats & oils, total added fats & oils, and total calories from added fats & oils and from all foods. Note: Due to the termination of select Current Industrial Reports (CIR) by the Census Bureau, data on some added fats and oils could not be updated beyond 2010 in the Food Availability Data System.

The pie charts below show the distribution of Calories among the different forms of added fats in the target year 1993 (chosen because it was within the Obesity Explosion), and in the year 2010, the last year full USDA data are available for added fats and oils.

Types of Added Fats and Oils Calories Consumed in 1993

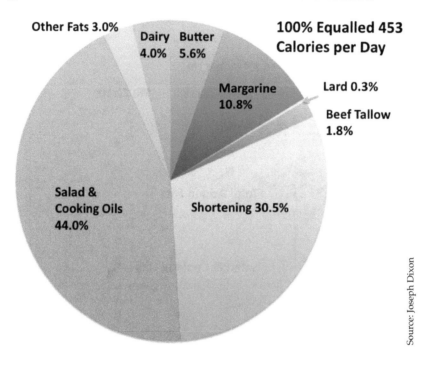

Other Fats 3.0%
Dairy 4.0%
Butter 5.6%
100% Equalled 453 Calories per Day
Margarine 10.8%
Lard 0.3%
Beef Tallow 1.8%
Salad & Cooking Oils 44.0%
Shortening 30.5%

Source: Joseph Dixon

Types of Added Fats and Oils Calories Consumed in 2010

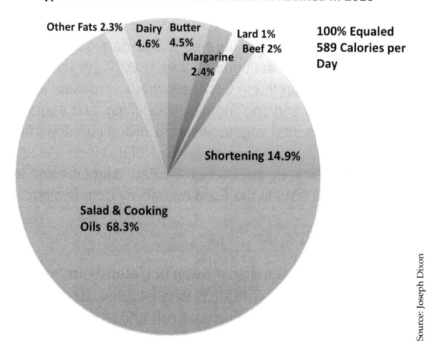

Other Fats 2.3%
Dairy 4.6%
Butter 4.5%
Lard 1%
Beef 2%
100% Equaled 589 Calories per Day
Margarine 2.4%
Shortening 14.9%
Salad & Cooking Oils 68.3%

Source: Joseph Dixon

For the 1993 pie chart for added fat and oils, the number one observation that can easily be made is that a great majority of Calories in added fats category came from vegetable oils that compose the salad and cooking oils (liquids) (light brown) and the shortening categories (solid fats) (blue). It is really quite amazing how little the other fats contribute to the Calories in our diet.

The 2010 pie chart for added fats and oils shows a stunning change in the distribution of Calories from the different fats. The Salad and Cooking oil category increased from 44.0% in 1993 to 68.3% in 2010. Therefore, the conclusions from the 2011 article by Blasbalg et al. would be even more pronounced today. That is, the fatty acid, linoleic acid (LA) (omega-6) intake would be even greater in 2010, and thus the omega-3 EPA and DHA intakes would be even more decreased in 2010.

Summary on the Consumption of Fats Leading Up to and during the Obesity Explosion

The Calorie intake and commodity statistics presented in this chapter reveal several major changes in Calorie consumption and the use of common food products. The changes that strikingly stand out are:

1. The decrease in the consumption of hard fats (butter, lard, margarine, and beef tallow) that started in the early 1960s was more than compensated for by the increases in the intake of soy oil and shortening. In fact, the increase in total added fats intake from 1980–2010 was about 250 Calories/person/day.

2. There was also a gradual increase in the consumption of chicken starting in the period after World War II. Consumption of chicken increased throughout the rest of the century. This change was probably the result of increases in availability of chicken as large chicken farms were established at this time. The feeding practices of these large farms led to chickens that contained greater fat per chicken. Of course, the composition of the chicken fat fatty acids also would have changed based upon the growing conditions and the feeds that were used to raise the chickens.

The large increase in the usage of soybean oil that started in the 1950s was the result of the adoption of soybeans by a large number of farmers in the U.S. after soybean cultivars were brought from China in the early 1900s. There was a delay of about 15 to 20 years from when farmers first started to grow soybeans until soybean products became widely available. Soybeans were first domesticated around

3,000 years ago, although the plant was known much earlier and grows wild all throughout China, Japan, Australia, and Papua New Guinea.[4]

In summary, when the observations from this chapter and the previous chapter are combined, the increases in per capita Calorie consumption over the past 30 to 40 years are largely due to increases in the consumption of three basic commodity groups.

1. Salad and cooking oil, driven by soybean and canola oils and other vegetable oils, by far increased the most over this period.
2. Corn and wheat flour both increased—probably because of the growth of the snack food industry.
3. Chicken consumption gradually increased over this whole period—probably as a result of fast-food restaurants and the increases in processed foods containing chicken.

The first commodity—vegetable oil, was no doubt required to cook or bake the other food commodities, corn and wheat products and chicken, that increased.

Interestingly, the per capita consumption of sugars stayed fairly consistent in the U.S. over the entire 1950 to 2000 period. This does not completely exonerate sugar as a causative factor of the Obesity Explosion. As will be discussed in the next chapter, the combination of sugar, sweeteners, fat, salt, and artificial and natural flavors would be responsible for the production of super palatable foods and desserts. When you go back to the beginning, humans have to consume more food per day in order for per capita Calorie intake to increase. This is not a chicken or the egg question.

---

[4] Shoemaker RC, Polzin KK, Lorenzen LL, Specht JE (1996). Molecular genetic mapping of soybean. In: *Soybeans: Genetics, Molecular Biology and Biotechnology.* pp. 37–56 (Edited by D.P. S. Verma and R.C. Shoemaker). Wallingford, UK: CAB International.

The Day Obesity was Born– The Birth of the Complex Artificial Flavor

When Precisely was Obesity Born?

We just discussed in the last two chapters how commodities changed in the 20th century. What else happened to the food we eat? It turns out that food companies started to put it all together. They learned what enticed people to eat. This was important to them. The more they sold the more money they made. So how did they do it—make food more desirable? Like so many discoveries, such as Einstein's Theory of Relativity, the Obesity Explosion was not born at one particular moment on one particular day. The scientific breakthroughs that ignited the Obesity Explosion, first needed to be synthesized as an idea, then expanded into a series of ideas, then into series of hypotheses, then into theories, then they were tested, just like in Edison's laboratory. The ideas were tried and worked on, and after many episodes of trial and error, possibly hundreds, in fact, they were finally made to work, and the era of the complex artificial flavors was born. The realization that humans reacted to complex artificial flavors was conveyed to a small group of industry experts, who then carried them forward to create usable products, until the state of the art was reached, and new foods that were never experienced before were sold in giant supermarkets. These new foods enriched the stockholders of these enormous companies. The realization that a series of chemicals could be mixed together to mimic, on many different levels, a near authentic taste or odor that humans would react to and desire, was a key, conceptual moment in the Obesity Explosion. A group of chemicals could provide a complex set of signals to the human brain that would plant the seed for the need to consume a particular food, whether it was previously wanted or needed. Human brains could now be manipulated by formulations that were designed by food chemists. Once these were added to bland packaged foods, they smashed the food intake regulatory system that was developed during evolution and refined during the 10,000 years of agriculture. Humans, walking around and partaking in their busy daily lives, were totally unaware of what was being developed in the laboratories of food companies, and once the products were introduced, they were powerless to resist. The laboratory discovery of the artificial complex flavor was the birth or the dawn of obesity, and was one of the most important components of the Obesity Explosion that rocked the Western world. This chapter tells how technological discoveries fed the Obesity Explosion.

Dr. David Kessler, a distinguish physician who was the Commissioner of the Food and Drug Administration, wrote a probing book concerning the Food Industry and how it has changed over the past 50 years.[1] Dr. Kessler is close to my Obesity Explosion heart. Like me, at times he had an irresistible desire for cookies—a concoction of sugar, fat, and flavors (hopefully chocolate), made into round disks that can vary between crunchy hard to squishy soft. Also like me, he has battled to keep his weight down most of his life.

Throughout his book, Dr. Kessler interviews people, friends, colleagues, as well as complete strangers, on how they eat in general, and why they are drawn to Calorie-dense foods such as cakes and cookies. One answer he received really struck me:[2]

> "Before I unwrapped the snacks, Maria said she had not been thinking of food, and she hadn't felt hungry. But now she felt compelled to stare at the cake and to imagine it in her mouth. She knew she wouldn't be able to resist for long. 'I keep looking at it,' she admitted. 'The outside coating is delicious. I'm fooling myself by thinking that I'll eat only one."
>
> Suddenly Maria became angry. 'I do not want them,' she said. 'But I cannot control my desire to eat them. I'm obsessing, I feel totally out of control.'"

Although Maria could not understand her desire, most likely the signals being sent around her brain were urging her to eat the snacks.

Then Dr. Kessler interviewed food company executives, as well as academic scientists, to learn the unwritten secrets of how food has been modified to make them super-palatable.

---

[1] Kessler DA (2009). The End of Overeating: Taking Control of the Insatiable American Appetite. New York: Rodale Inc.

[2] Kessler DA (2009). Ibid, p. 25.

Dr. Kessler interviewed Jerilyn Brusseau, one of the founders of Cinnabon, and she told him the story of how the successful food chain was established.[3]

Cinnabon, a chain of small pocket bakeries that sell a delicious, gooey cinnamon roll, got its start in the kitchen of Jerilyn Brusseau, in the suburbs of Seattle. She started a small café-bakery that became very well known for her tasty cinnamon rolls. An entrepreneur from the restaurant sector called her up and proposed they team up. Together they established what has now become a chain of hundreds of Cinnabon bakeries across America. After so much success with her rolls, Dr. Kessler was lucky enough to get her to describe some of the components that went into her irresistible cinnamon rolls. A summary of her description gives clues to why Cinnabons are so good, and possibly irresistible. They have the following: a soft dough center that is chewy yet smooth; highly selected cinnamon (from Vietnam) caramel in the center; three kinds of sugar—granular, brown, and powder—used in different places in the roll; and a frosting made from cream cheese. Some other ingredients are salt and lemon. I have eaten Cinnabons maybe 10 times in my life— usually in an airport. The rumor is that they pump Cinnabon aroma into the food court. They are absolutely delicious and tasty, and possibly irresistible. Therefore, I decided never to walk into a Cinnabon shop again. I believed that I could become very attached to them, and I wanted to prevent such an association.

When it comes to being confronted with delicious foods, there are things about them that we would never recognize unless we were told by a food chemist. Dr. Kessler had an extensive discussion with food scientist, Gail Vance Civille. She told Dr. Kessler about the process of caramelizing food. Here is the short exchange between them:[4]

"'What else produces the sensory hits we like?' I asked.

'Caramelizing food—the process of browning starches, sugars, and proteins—helps do this, she said. Caramelization generates sweeter aromatics and gives food 'more impact, more volatiles.' It's a flavor found in many foods we produce in this country.'"

"It's a key driving of liking"

'Absolutely. On a sweet product it's often the number one driver.'"

Gail Vance Civille also commented about what fat adds to food. As a lipid biochemist, I am well aware of how fat contributes to the taste of foods. But it is wonderful to hear a food chemist describe it.

---

[3] Kessler DA (2009). Ibid, p. 74.

[4] Kessler DA (2009). Ibid, p. 89.

Here is another exchange with Dr. Kessler[5]:

Dr. Kessler: "'Tell me how fat engages the senses. Why does the industry add so much of it to food?'

'One reason, she responded, is that fat contributes to texture in many ways, giving food body, crunch, creaminess, or contrast. Fat makes food feel thicker and richer and "will contribute to a sense of fullness in the mouth."'

'It also promoted the release of flavor-enhancing chemicals…'

'Also, fat helps flavors merge and meld, creating a smooth sensation as it brings disparate ingredients together in a symphonic whole.'

"Fat contributes to a smooth, even bolus (the wad that forms as you chew food) in the mouth. If fat is removed from a product, it won't break down the same way. Rather than melting, 'You get little tiny globs of stuff suspended in saliva,' she said. Civille didn't have to add that this would make for an unpleasant sensory experience."

"Fat also lingers after we swallow food, leaving flavor behind in the mouth. 'Unlike bad wine that just falls off, the volatility is still there, so you still have pleasurable aftertaste.'"

Dr. Kessler's book is full of other insights into how the food industry won the battle of getting a wide swath of people to just keep eating.

Michael Moss' Explosive Book, "Salt Sugar Fat: How the Food Giants Hooked Us"

Food companies have made significant discoveries concerning what makes humans crave certain foods. Another investigator of the food industry is Michael Moss, who was an investigative reporter for The New York Times. He won a Pulitzer Prize in 2010 for his reporting concerning the meat industry. I first learned of Mr. Moss when I read his article, "The Extraordinary Science of Addictive Junk Food," published February 20, 2013 in the New York Times Magazine.[6] This article was adapted from "Salt Sugar Fat: How the Food Giants Hooked Us," published in 2013 by Random House.[7] I went on to read his excellent book, and later he gave a lecture at Rutgers University.

---

[5] Kessler DA (2009). Ibid, pp. 89–90.

[6] http://www.nytimes.com/2013/02/24/magazine/the-extraordinary-science-of-junk-food.html

[7] Moss M (2014, paperback). *Salt Sugar Fat: How the Food Giants Hooked Us*. New York: Random House Trade Paperbacks.

Here is short summary of Mr. Moss' article: What makes this article, and the book from which it was excerpted, so powerful is that Mr. Moss was able to obtain documents that support his entire story. Michael Moss stated, "What I found, over four years of research and reporting, was a conscious effort—taking place in labs and marketing meetings and grocery-store aisles—to get people hooked on foods that are convenient and inexpensive." Mr. Moss interviewed over 300 people who had been involved, or are still involved, with the food industry. In this article, he relays examples of how certain foods were formulated to make products irresistible to consumers. Foods that he mentioned in the magazine article were Dr. Pepper, Prego spaghetti sauce, fully packaged Lunchables with dessert, the line extension of Lay's potato chips, and several other major processed foods we all know and unfortunately, love.

Mr. Moss's article begins with a recap of a one-day meeting of major food executives in 1999. In a presentation by a vice president of Kraft, named Michael Mudd, it was posited that the high rates of childhood and adult obesity were in part due to products supplied by the major food companies. Mr. Mudd suggested that one way to combat obesity included lowering salt, fat, and sugar in their products, and pulling back on their advertising of packaged and front line food products. This presentation sounded very positive concerning the health of Americans. But it wasn't going to last. Later in the same meeting, Stephen Sanger, CEO of General Mills, indicated that General Mills would not change course, and that he would not alter recipes that had been formulated to be successful. The possibility that major food companies would do their part to fight the Obesity Explosion was definitely deflated in this meeting.

Here are some major food products that Mr. Moss discussed in his article:

For Dr. Pepper, Moss saw the report where Howard Moskowitz, a food industry consultant, detailed how to increase the acceptance of Dr. Pepper by consumers. He even cited specific pages in the report where Moskowitz described by reformulation how to increase the allure of Dr. Pepper. We learned that in Prego spaghetti sauce, after tomatoes, sugar was made the next greatest ingredient so as to lure consumers. I remember explicitly when my family first tried Prego spaghetti sauce, the sweetness was mind boggling. However, everyone in the family, including me, liked it. We used it for a while and then went on to another tomato sauce. Another extremely revealing story was about the grandchildren of Bob Drane, the man who invented Lunchables. Drane's daughter was of a different philosophy than her father. She wanted her family to "eat very healthfully." Therefore, his grandchildren were not allowed to eat Lunchables for school lunch.

Mr. Moss discusses an interesting strategy in the food industry that most of us who spend time in major supermarkets will be aware of, this is the line extension, where products such as the original Oreos have morphed into over 30 different "Oreo" varieties. The possibility of finding that perfect Oreo that could wow almost every possible palate was enhanced many fold by giving shoppers many more choices within the product!

In the case of potato chips, food industry scientists again followed the food industry's very effective strategy (line extension) to increase the sales of well-known products. In this case, the classic Lay's potato chip brand was extended to include product cousins such as chips with salt & vinegar, salt & pepper, cheddar, and sour cream flavoring. In a later chapter, "Growing Up before Obesity," I write about how the local small grocery store one block from my house in Brooklyn, NY, carried just one kind of potato chip in the late 50s and early 60s. The brand was Wise Potato Chips. I still remember the precise taste of this potato chip. Mr. Moss also described how Frito-Lay executives had hoped to develop "designer sodium," one day. Such a super sodium could possibly decrease the actual milligrams of sodium in their products by a considerable amount. This would save Frito-Lay from the critics who pointed to the sodium in their snacks.

An interview of Michael Moss conducted by Ms. Johannah Sakimura, RD, one of the students in my obesity class, can be viewed at: http://www.everydayhealth.com/weight/unholy-trinity-behind-junk-food-michael-moss.aspx

The Day the Obesity Explosion was Ignited—The Birth of the Artificial Complex Flavor

In his book, "The Dorito Effect," author Mark Schatzker,[8] tells the story of Arch West, a vice president at the Frito-Lay Company, who in the early 1960s came up with the idea to introduce tortilla chips, a new snack, into the American market. He named them "Doritos," a Mexican word that translates as, "little pieces of gold." Up until this time, Frito-Lay made mainly potato chips, and one could only eat something resembling a tortilla in a Mexican styled restaurant in the far southern areas of the U.S. He convinced his superiors at Frito-Lay to try the new product, and Doritos were introduced in the U.S. in 1964. The first Doritos were primarily plain salted toasted corn chips, and they were a total flop. Sales went nowhere. So Arch West went back to the drawing board and worked with technologists at Frito-Lay to develop a taco-flavored corn chip. When this version of Doritos hit the market, it was a resounding success with the American public. And the American public was never the same.

By 2010 there were more than a dozen different flavored Doritos on the market, including my favorite, Nacho Cheese. The success of Doritos spurred other companies to develop similar tortilla chip products, and many other highly flavored snack

---

[8] Schatzker M (2015). *The Dorito Effect: The Surprising New Truth About Food and Flavor.* New York: Simon & Schuster.

foods. Today, one can walk down a very long, full aisle of these snack foods in their local supermarket (Corn intake has increased during the past 50 years).

Another story[9] Mark Schatzker tells is the story of why and how McCormick and Company (the spice company) developed Imitation Vanilla. After the plantations growing vanilla beans were destroyed during a civil war in Madagascar in the 1970s, the price of natural vanilla extract went sky high. (By the way, the price of vanilla has again increased in 2018 due to a powerful cyclone that hit Madagascar[10]). McCormick directed its analytical department to develop a suitable alternative to authentic vanilla extract. At first it was difficult to obtain a reasonable authentic vanilla taste and aroma. Then one day in the late 1970s, lab technician Marianne Gillette was running vanilla extract through a gas chromatograph, and in addition to using the instrument's detector to monitor the individual chemicals coming through, she was smelling the peaks (component chemicals) as they were swept out of the instrument. In this way she discovered a strong scent in authentic vanilla extract that was actually from a very small peak in the chromatogram (signifying a compound in very low concentration). The chemical compound that she smelled coming off the column in this small peak was very potent, but because of its low amount, it had been missed in earlier analyses. Marianne Gillette's highly sensitive sense of smell led her to a giant discovery. What Ms. Gillette had discovered was one of the critical ingredients in natural vanilla extract that was important for its overall flavor/aroma. This one discovery allowed McCormick to go on and develop their Imitation Vanilla product, which was put on the market in 1982, and since then, has been very successful and profitable. The take home message from this story was—who needs the raw plant? Because now it was possible to recreate the important flavors and aromas in vanilla through chemistry. The artificial complex chemical flavor was born, and so the fuse for the Obesity Explosion was lit and the bomb exploded.

Did the Food Companies Have a Secret Ally in Their Efforts to Make Foods Irresistible?

If you read Chandler Burr's book,[11] "The Emperor of Scent," he tells the story of Dr. Luca Turin, who is a rather unique, loose cannon scientist in the field of the sense of smell, or as the scientists themselves call it, sensory science. The book is also about

---

[9] Schatzker M (2015). Ibid, p. 47.

[10] See: https://www.theguardian.com/money/2018/aug/27/one-in-five-vanilla-ice-creams-has-no-vanilla-cream-or-fresh-milk. Accessed August 29, 2018.

[11] Burr C (2002). *The Emperor of Scent: A Story of Perfume, Obsession, and the Last Mystery of the Senses*. Random House Publishing Group. Kindle Edition.

the fragrance industry, which uses organic chemistry to develop and produce thousands of fragrances and flavors. The olfactory system in humans is one of the most complex communications systems in the body. It is involved in sex, mother–child bonding, finding safe foods, and bringing joy when one walks through a beautiful garden. Mr. Burr beautifully explained that the purpose of the olfactory system for early humans was to find nutritious and safe foods. The hunter–gatherers didn't have food labels or expiration dates to determine how safe the food was. One generation passed vital information about nutrition and foods to the next generation, and then they too developed a sensitive sense of smell that helped avoid toxic plant foods. A fairly recent review of the olfactory system is presented in an article by Silva Teixeira et al.[12]

Besides writing about Luca Turin and the power of the olfactory system, Chandler Burr also wrote about the "Big Boys," who are the major companies that fly beneath the radar and produce secretive and powerful scents. Mr. Burr writes[13]:

> "Virtually all the smells in all scented products in the world are manufactured by seven huge companies that operate in carefully guarded anonymity: International Flavors & Fragrances (United States), Givaudan Roure (Switzerland), Quest International (Britain), Firmenich (Switzerland), Haarmann & Reimer (Germany), Dragoco (Germany), and Takasago (Japan). These are the Big Boys, the industrial giants of the production and sale of a specific, unusual product: molecules.

> "Molecules that trigger the human sense of taste and, above all, the sense of smell. Taste is, actually, a dwarfish, minimally functional sense responding to only six different stimuli: sweet, sour, salt, bitter, umami (richness), and astringent; smell—which in point of fact gives us some 90 percent of what we taste—is thought to respond to ten thousand or so distinguishable molecular smells, but we only say ten thousand because (and this is literally true) we've thus far never touched the limits of smell's power to detect odorant molecules. The Big Boys' molecules generate roughly $ 20 billion a year in economic activity. They employ hundreds of chemists, molecular jockeys who spend their days welding atoms together to create new molecules with new smells. And, upstairs, they employ an army of perfumers, who spend their days mixing these molecules into new scented elixirs."

[12] Silva Teixeira CS, Cerqueira NM, Silva Ferreira AC (2016). Unravelling the olfactory sense: From the gene to odor perception. *Chem Senses* 41(2):105–121. https://www.ncbi.nlm.nih.gov/pubmed/26688501

[13] Burr C (2002). Ibid, pp. 56–57.

These giant companies, which manufacture fragrances—also manufacture flavors. And they virtually have produced thousands of flavors to choose from.

Through the activities described above, the American public would henceforth be subjected to snacks and foods that would be formulated to be irresistible, and once one started to eat them, it would be almost impossible to stop eating at a reasonable amount.

Many of these discoveries, many of which were mainly missed by the main scientific community, have led to a significant dampening of the energy/weight regulatory system that had worked perfectly fine in humans for at least 200,000 years, and which worked especially well during the past 10,000 years of agriculture. The result was the Obesity Explosion, which became noticeable around the year 1980, and which continues today.

Up until "The Day Obesity Was Born," many changes in society had made everyday life much different than experienced before. But after this day, the genie was out of the "bliss" bottle, and thereafter, a majority of humans found it difficult to stop eating. The precipitous increase in body weight among Americans over the past 40 years has been nothing less than extraordinary. All the changes in foods and in the fabric of our culture, with special note for the rise of the automobile and the digital revolution, certainly contributed to the assault on our ability to maintain body weight. But something else was needed (a searing discovery of some sort) to tip the tide in favor of losing control of body weight—the proverbial "straw that broke the camel's back." The laboratory discovery of the artificial complex flavor was the birth or dawn of the Obesity Explosion. Afterwards, whether they wanted to or not, Americans continued to eat after they consumed a normal amount of food. This chapter reviewed four books that tell the story of what happened to break the camel's back. These books described the beginning of the birth of the modern complex artificial chemical flavor, or, another way to describe it: the birth of the Age of the Super Intense Taste/Aroma—or the Age of Imitation Foods!

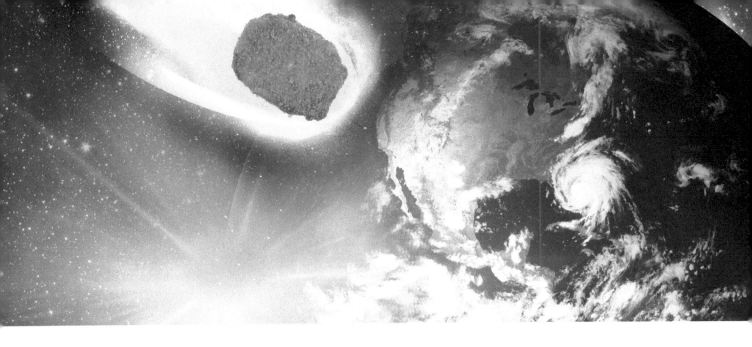

PART 3

Yesterday and Today: How America Changed During the 20th Century—Obesity and Modern Culture

Growing Up Before the Obesity Explosion

What was it like to be a child before the Obesity Explosion? All throughout this book I present many of the changes in our society that have contributed to the onset of obesity in the United States. Since I grew up in the two decades before the Obesity Explosion, I can tell you. My overall conclusion is that it was just as rich a time to grow up as today, when we have a more technological based culture. In fact, I feel bad for kids who stay inside for long periods of time to play video games. It was not something a Hunter–gatherer kid would do. And it wasn't something I did when I was a kid in the 1960s. I played outside from morning to night in the summer, and sometimes in the winter too!

Grocery Shopping Before Obesity

I remember many things about my early life in Brooklyn, NY, that pointed to a very active childhood. One example is that my mother did not drive, and therefore, when we went to the supermarket, we took out the grocery cart and pulled it behind us. We needed to walk 2 and ½ flat blocks and then we headed down a long steep hill. I hated walking down that hill, because I knew that later on, we would need to walk back up it. We walked another three blocks and came to our local A&P supermarket. We went in, attached our cart to the small grocery push cart, and then proceeded to go down the first short aisle on the left side of the store (I can still visualize the layout). At the rear was a small open top freezer that held the ice cream and ices. We then moved to the next aisle, which was much longer. After grabbing groceries from the middle aisle, we went all the way to the rear of the store to cross over to the third aisle.

After making the turn, you then went down the final long third aisle to the checkout counters. That was it—three aisles in all! The A&P was stocked with staples but with little else. This small A&P had a dairy section, a bakery section, a small frozen food section, a canned goods section, but few others—not the dozens of sections that are found in modern mega supermarkets today. And one type of item our small A&P had very little of were processed foods. But it did have the essentials.

One of my greatest fears as a child (I still have dreams about this even today!) was being asked by my mother to go back and get something that we had forgotten to put into the grocery cart. I could not go back up the last aisle we had come down because the flow of traffic was only one way and I would be run over by the other shoppers. So I needed to slip under the bar that separated the checkouts from the first aisle and then I would navigate back through the entire store to get the needed item. I then needed to go to the third aisle and weave through the shoppers with their push carts to get back to the check out. The smallness of the A&P made only one-way traffic possible. After paying we would load the brown bags into our 2-wheel pull cart and start the walk back home. And yes, we needed to climb that long hill to get there. I will always remember the pain of going up that hill as a little boy!

Having a Child Help Make the Family Meal at Home

Today as I write this in 2020, it has been reported by several researchers that currently 40% to 50% of money spent on food is spent eating outside the home (I will present this data in a later chapter). This is an astonishing figure because as a child growing up, my family went out to eat infrequently—maybe twice a year. And usually this was for a very special occasion, such as a birthday or graduation. We essentially never went out to eat in a restaurant. No one that I knew at the time did. From this we can infer some basic facts. First, when I was a child in the late 50s and early 60s, at least where I lived, most food was consumed in the home, and therefore, most food was prepared in the home.

In order for this to occur a parent needed to be at home in order to shop, prepare, and serve the meals. When I was young, this was my mother, who did not work outside the home (she typed invoices and correspondence for my father, who had his own business). And this was possible because the economic paradigm at the time allowed for one wage earner to support a family, and this allowed one spouse to remain at home.

This basic operational model had other major effects on family life. Since a spousal unit was always at home, the smaller kids could be watched by a parent and taken along on errands and visits around the neighborhood. Being home, a child could help the parent in the kitchen with elementary tasks. This was an excellent opportunity to learn how to cook at a very young age. In an extended analogy, this was not unlike a child following around a mother or father to learn how to gather and prepare food in a Hunter–Gatherers' village.

If a child in a village can learn helpful family tasks, why not a child in a modern American home? In fact, this was how I learned to cook, and probably where I carried out my first chemistry experiments. From a very early age I knew how to wash vegetables, peel potatoes, mix ingredients in a bowl, and prepare meats. I was also the person who set the table and put drinks from the refrigerator on the table. After doing this many times—it becomes second nature, like learning a language. When I later went to college it turned out to be an essential survival skill to make meals in my apartment. And like learning to ride a bike, cooking is something that you never forget how to do.

One food I loved to prepare and was in fact the "principal starch" of our family was potatoes. My mother made potatoes in every conceivable way—baked, boiled, mashed, french fried from scratch, au gratin, broiled, and as an ingredient of hash (mixed with meat). So my whole life I have made homemade potatoes an important part of my diet.

Shopping in Manhattan Before the Shopping Mall

When my mother took me with her on a shopping trip for clothes, it was an opportunity to eat outside the house, but not at a fast-food restaurant, because they did not really exist at the time. My mother would take me with her on the subway into New York City (aka Manhattan). She would shop in midtown at Macy's or Gimbel's near Herald Square. Usually we ate in a department store cafeteria. But occasionally, we ate at the Horn & Hardart Automat in midtown. The Automat was a flashy, bright cafeteria style restaurant where there was a large sitting area surrounded on two sides by long walls containing hundreds of shiny aluminum doors (12 in wide, 8 in high) with little windows through which you could see the foods. It reminded me of how the crew of the U.S.S. Enterprise on the 1960s version of the television show "Star Trek" obtained their food on the cafeteria deck.

This was such an amazing experience and I always wondered whether there were robots behind those little doors and in the back that made the food. Actually there were hard working food service workers loading the compartments with food but we couldn't see them. My mother gave me the coins to put into the slots, and after putting the money in, you turned a knob and then you could open the door and take out the dish with the food. I would eat the baked beans or the macaroni and cheese, both standards at the Automat. My mother would always eat the creamed spinach or a fish cake. These were relatively small one-course meals.

The trip to the Automat made the long subway ride and walking through crowds and busy traffic of Manhattan streets somewhat bearable. At least there was something exciting to look forward to while my mother shopped. And my feet would hurt and sweat the entire time. I can still feel them! After the trip to the store and lunch, we headed back home on the subway.

I would fall asleep to the back and forth sway of the subway cars. Right before our stop, my mother would wake me up and then we climbed our way to the street where we would find ourselves near the A&P supermarket I described earlier. Once on the sidewalk we walked back to our house, walking up the same hill that I dreaded when going to the A&P. Finally, we were home!

How was that trip into Manhattan on the subway different than the trip to the mall by car today? We walked at least a half-mile from our house to the subway stop. After descending the stairs we needed to wait for the train. In Manhattan we had to walk up the stairs to the street and then we walked to Herald Square from 6th Avenue. And on the way back everything was reversed. Today, in most cases, people drive to the mall, park their cars, and walk in. They shop for several hours, about the same amount of time as we rummaged up and down several department stores on our shopping trip. Today the modern shopper walks through the mall but does not exercise anywhere near as much as we did taking the subway. People may stop and eat fast food at the food court. After they are through, they walk a short distance to their cars, get in and drive home, where they park in the driveway. Our shopping and eating experiences in Manhattan were much different than those experienced by shoppers at the modern mall of today.

By eating in a Department store cafeteria we obtained basic food to eat and it did not consist of a burger and fries or another popular fast food. Some common cafeteria foods at the time were a sandwich on toast, tuna fish on a green leaf salad, soup and crackers, a meat with vegetable entree, and don't forget a bowl of Jello or pudding for dessert. Drinks were only 8 oz at most. Who would want to drink a 20 oz drink? Unthinkable! We were used to eating small-sized meals for relatively normal-sized people (as least 95% of us were normal-sized back then!).

Once home, my mother would start supper, and I would help her. We would eat dinner at home like we did every other night. But it was certainly a treat to eat in a cafeteria or at the Automat. My mother and I did eat out, but we also had walked a great deal during the day, and we walked down and up that monstrous hill, and we burned up a lot of kilocalories doing it.

The One Exception—Brooklyn Pizza

There was one exception to our usual experience of eating meals at home. If I am to be honest, we did spend money on food made outside the home. After all, Brooklyn pizza is famous throughout the U.S. Every so often when my mother needed a break, we would order pizza or two from the local pizzeria. We would call in our order and my father would drive and pick the pizza pies up from the pizzeria. This was always a treat for us. Also, on some occasions, when I was older, and out at night at the boys club meeting where we did calisthenics, I would stop on the way home at a pizza place to get a slice. I remember that the price of a slice of pizza was 15 cents. And I remember quite vividly that the price of a ride on the NYC subway was always the same price as a slice of pizza. At the time it was also 15 cents for a ride on the subway. Today in 2020 the price of the subway is $2.75 and the slice of pizza runs from $3.00 to $5.00 depending on the location of the pizza shop. So the equivalency relationship between a slice of pizza and the cost of a subway ride is holding up pretty well.

My First Hamburger Fast-Food Experience

There were very few fast-food restaurants in Brooklyn at the time. It was in the summer of 1969 and some of my older friends were going to the Woodstock Music and Art Fair in upstate New York. I asked my mother if I could go with them. She said definitely not. After all, I was only 15 years old and I had only 1 year of high school behind me. Unknown to me, my mother had a better idea—I was to fly down to Atlanta Georgia and spend a week with my two sisters, Rita and Jeanne. This trip coincided exactly with Woodstock. So I flew down to Georgia, and I really do not have many memories of the trip. However, the one thing that I do remember perfectly is walking across the street from Rita's apartment and eating a Whopper sandwich at a Burger King fast-food restaurant.

The experience is indelibly etched into my unprepared mind (most likely there are specific neurons that hold this memory!). The charcoal broiled burger, the lettuce, tomato, pickle, and ketchup. And the mayo on the lettuce. All packed into a sesame seed bun. How delicious. High salt, high fat, and I am sure there is sugar somewhere in the concoction (indeed, the bun was made from highly refined wheat flour with a high Glycemic Index). The combination of flavors was a taste orgy to my brain. To this day, I remember that experience, and sometimes at the craziest times, I crave a Whopper sandwich. At a moment's notice, I will be driven to go out and find a Burger King fast-food restaurant. So there was something in that sandwich that caused a pathway of neurons to be laid down in my brain. And whenever there is activity in that pathway of neurons, I need to go out and find a Whopper burger to eat! Nothing else will satisfy me. It reminds me of a Hunter–Gatherer getting up from his camp fire to go stalk an antelope! Well, not exactly.

Some of my friends made it to Woodstock, and some didn't. For sure I did not get to attend the once in a lifetime festival. There is no doubt that my mother out-smarted me.

Playing Outside on the Street Before Obesity

A few years ago I caught a wonderful program on Public Television entitled, "New York Street Games."[1] This program consisted of older New Yorkers, including some celebrities, remembering all the different street games that they use to play outside on the streets when they were growing up in New York City. And the funny thing about it was that as each new game was mentioned on the program, I jumped up and yelled, "I played that!" In the early 60s, there was nothing to do inside the house or apartment except to get into some kind of trouble. So whenever possible, no matter what the weather, you went outside and tried to hook up with your friends. I'm mainly talking about my elementary school years—so maybe ages 9 to 14. I would go outside and always walk about one to two blocks to the place where my friends usually hung out. And if your friends were not around, you went around and rang doorbells until someone came outside. After sitting around for a few minutes, we threw out all sorts of ideas about what games we were going to play. These included a long list of games, including: all sorts of versions of tag, ringolevio, stoop ball, stickball, slap ball, and basic rough housing in general. It always helped to have a series of one car garages (say three in a row) right there on the block where you could play one of the ball games. And of course, all of these games used a small pink, bouncy rubber ball called a "Spaldeen." (Actually, a small ball produced by Spalding, the well-known maker of basketballs and footballs.) If during the course of a game one of these balls went over the garages or rolled into the sewer, you had to go buy another one. Luckily, there was a small candy store half a block away that sold them. I must have bought a hundred of these balls over the course of my childhood. We also played Johnny on the pony against the garages. We also played bottle caps (Skully), where a square field of play was drawn on the street with chalk, and we brought our own bottle caps that were usually filled in with some kind of putty to make them a little heavier than normal. You would use your thumb and index finger to flick the bottle cap between the little corner safe zones. And although totally politically incorrect at the current time, we used to play army with our own plastic play guns. I especially was fond of my "Man from Uncle" spy pistol. The cars parked on the street were especially good for hiding behind or even under. For stick ball, you usually played right in the middle of the street, with parked cars are both sides of the street. The streets we hung out on were side streets, and there were less cars in those days, so we might have to stop playing every 3 or 4 minutes to let a car pass by. There were two versions of stick ball—if you had enough guys—you could have two teams of three or four and use bases drawn on the street with chalk. But if you didn't have enough players, there was an individual version where you needed to hit the

---

[1] https://en.wikipedia.org/wiki/New_York_Street_Games

ball straight and see how far the ball would go (meaning, how many round sewer covers the ball would pass). And of course, we might walk several block over to the fully cement-surfaced playground to play basketball or soft ball in the dedicated courts and fields. If you wish to hear about the games we played on the streets and sidewalks, definitely try to watch the documentary listed above.

One very interesting thing about the above play activities was that they were never, and I mean never, supervised by a parent. Of course, parents (usually mothers) would stick their heads out a door or window to check on us, but I never once remember a parent being with us as we played our games. It just seemed to be a group dynamic where we looked out after ourselves, and we were very aware of where we were and who to hang out with and who not to hang out with. I personally was not very good at sitting on a stoop and doing nothing, so we either played a game, or we went wandering around the neighborhood. If I became really bored, I went home, and usually helped by mother around the house!

Running an Errand to the Corner Grocery Store

Quite often my mother would send me to Oscar's Deli for one or two items that we needed right away. Oscar's Deli, which was around the corner and one block away, was a typical corner "Mom and Pop" deli (now often called a Bodaega, or the corner Asian market) in Brooklyn at the time (1960s). You would go there to get a container of milk or a loaf of bread, or even some deli meats and sliced cheese. Oscar's was always busy as many people in the neighborhood did not have cars and the A&P grocery store was at least a 30-minute walk away.

One of the things that I would occasionally buy at Oscar's was a bag of potato chips that my mother wanted for us as a treat. I can still remember their exact location in his store—in a small rack just near the entrance. What was so different back then was that there was <u>only</u> one brand of potato chips sold at Oscar's and at the local A&P—it was Wise Potato Chips, and of course they came in two basic sizes—large and small. Anyone who has tasted Wise Potato Chips knows that they have a fairly distinctive greasy taste to them. And to the Wise company's credit, they taste exactly the same today as they did 55 years ago! The taste is precisely hard wired into my brain! Today if there was a contest, I could pick a Wise potato chip out of the 30 or so common brands.

Now contrast the potato chip and snack foodscape today with what it was back then. I recently went into a large grocery store near where I live and took note of where the snack foods were. First, there was a whole display of snack foods in the front of the store just as you came in the main doors. Then if you searched the aisles— there was a complete aisle, from the very front of the store to the rear of the store, displaying every type of snack food one could possibly desire. There are so many different brands of potato chips and several different flavors within each brand, that it is indeed almost difficult to choose the one want to buy. But certainly, the average American consumer will find something in that aisle that, once the bag or box was opened, would be so addictive that it would be difficult to stop eating.

A recent article reported on a study where "'dietary variability" (the role played by having many versions of the same food) influenced the consumption of Calories.[2] The availability of "...71 different types of pepperoni pizza across 14 brands..." in the United Kingdom "was associated with compromised controls of food intake." So maybe having a limited amount of healthy choices (as was the case in our small A&P market) was important in maintaining healthy weights across a wide range of the population in the time before the Obesity Explosion.

---

[2] Hardman CA, Ferriday D, Kyle L, Rogers PJ, Brunstrom JM (2015). So many brands and varieties to choose from: Does this compromise the control of food intake in humans? *PLoS One* 10(4):e0125869 https://www.ncbi.nlm.nih.gov/pubmed/25923118

Americans in the 1960s Before the Obesity Explosion

Here is another trip back in time showing what life was like when I was growing up. The previous chapter covered from when I was 5 to 7 years old up to about 15 years old. In my mid-teens it was the late 1960s, and I remember it well. I graduated high school in 1972 and then went to college. How does that time compare with how teenagers and college students live today? We can't go back 10,000 years ago, or even 1,000 years ago, and see what people looked like in terms of body weight. For one thing, no matter what their body weight was at the time, the humans then were much unhealthier than humans are today, and their life expectancy was extremely short (about an average of 30 years of age). But if you wish to go back and see a population that was much thinner than Americans are today, all you need to do is take a time machine or a DeLorean DMC-12 back to the 1960s in the United States. People were much thinner then.

If you wish to relive the 1960s, or you are too young and wish to see the 1960s for the first time, and you don't have a time machine or a DeLorean, an easy way to go back is to look at the movie "Woodstock" on YouTube (turn down the sound if you do not like rock and roll!; also, don't look too closely if you are upset by nudity, even if it is for science!). You will absolutely be amazed how thin teenagers and young adults were back in the 1960s. Of course, you will see some heavy people, too (but very few—possibly close to the historic 4% in the population), as there have been heavy people in all generations (probably because having heavy individuals in the tribe was an important evolutionary survival mechanism). The following is one photo out of many on the Internet of the Woodstock Music and Art Festival, held in White Lake, New York on August 15 to 18, 1969. This photograph is one of my favorites because we visit the town of Woodstock, NY, every summer and we love to swim in swimming holes, which are fed by creeks from the local mountains. But to get the full effect, you must go look at the movie to see young people in 1969!

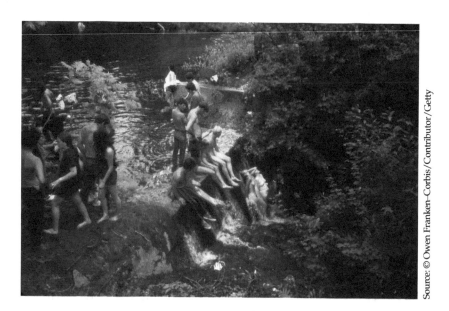

Source: © Owen Franken-Corbis/Contributor/Getty

Go look at the movie, "Woodstock" on YouTube if you wish to see the thinness of young adults in 1969! It is amazing!

About 500,000 people made it to Woodstock, and many more tried to go but did not make it because the highways and roads to the festival became completely blocked with cars. I asked my mother if I could go, and the answer was a resounding "no."

As someone who was very heavy as a child (until about the age of 16), I was happy to find this photograph of me when I was in college. The photograph shows my roommates and me in our senior year (1976) of college at SUNY-Binghamton.[1]

Senior Year, SUNY-Binghamton, 1976

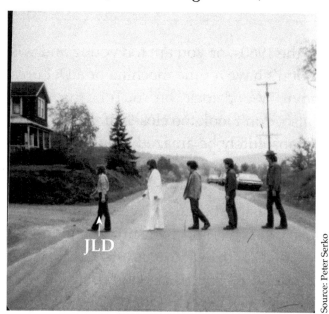

JLD

Source: Peter Serko

---

[1] Photograph by Peter Serko, May 1976. https://peterserko.com

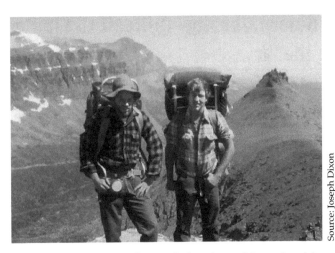

Source: Joseph Dixon

The author (right) and backpacking buddy (Thomas Kane) in an old fashioned selfie (using timer) taken in Glacier National Park, summer 1975. Photograph by Joseph L. Dixon.

We are outside of our house reenacting a famous album cover. I am the first in line and I was thin through the last portion of high school and all through college because I changed my eating habits and became very active, including backpacking for 2 months throughout the entire western U.S. when I was just 20 years old (see next photograph). The training for the backpacking trips involved running at college and in Prospect Park in Brooklyn.

Life Before Computers and Obesity

Because computers and ubiquitous fast food were not yet available, what was life like as a high school or college student in the 1960s through the early 1970s?

Although I did not make it to the Woodstock Music and Art Festival in August of 1969, I remember life at that time and how different it was from today. I was 15 years old in the summer of 1969 and still in high school. I lived in Brooklyn, New York, and city life was all I knew. In order to go to high school in the morning, I walked three long blocks up a steep hill and caught a bus that traveled along Seventh Avenue (Called Park Slope—now one of the trendiest neighborhoods in revitalized Brooklyn) to Flatbush Avenue, where I transferred to a subway for the remaining trip to Crown Heights in Brooklyn. If I was lucky, I made it to my high school in about an hour (usually it took an hour and a half). And after school in the afternoon, I often walked home through Prospect Park, which also took about an hour. Often, I stayed after school to play basketball in the gym. But it was important to make it home to have dinner with my mother and father, and whomever of my siblings was home at time.

Driving to College Before Obesity—Difficult to Find a Place to Eat along the Way

After I graduated from high school, I went to college in upstate New York. This was my first time away from home and it took some time to get used to living in a dorm room with a roommate. But there was no doubt that I loved being away at college. Once a week I tried to call home, usually on the weekend. There was one telephone booth in the lobby on the ground floor of the dormitory, and if you did not wish to wait on a long line, you needed to get up early on a Saturday morning to make a call. There were no private telephones or cell phones. We couldn't even imagine having a cell phone.

After trips back home or at the beginning of a semester, I would drive up to college either with a friend, or later on by myself when I had a car.

When it was time to drive back to college I packed the car and took off about 10 a.m. I was driving from Brooklyn to Binghamton NY, and I had eaten breakfast but probably did not pack a lunch. After navigating the bridges and roads out of New York City, I was on the NY State Thruway and would soon take Route 17 to head northwest to Binghamton. It was getting near 12 noon and I was a little hungry. I just put it out of my mind and made a note to stop at the Roscoe diner in about an hour. The traffic was fairly light and I made good time. I exited at Roscoe and pulled into the Roscoe diner's parking lot. It was packed and I knew immediately it would be a long wait to get seated and then eat lunch.

I walked in and when I heard it would be a 40-minute wait before I could sit down, I just turned around and got back into the car. I put my hunger away and continued on my trip to Binghamton. Actually, being hungry keeps you awake and alert while you drive. There is nothing more sleep inducing than eating a big lunch. Several hours later I arrived at my apartment in Endicott, NY (close to SUNY-Binghamton). I looked in the refrigerator and observed a few very suspect food items in there. So I had to walk down to the local grocery to buy some milk, bread, and cheese. I made myself a sandwich and drank some milk. I was finally not hungry—it wasn't a big deal. It was 1974 and it was typical to make the drive between New York City and Binghamton without eating. After all, there were very few places to eat along the way. There were certainly no fast-food places to stop—at least none that I can remember. And not seeing a restaurant at every exit didn't coax me into stopping and eating. Not having an easy place to stop and eat was very common at this time before the appearance of the obesogenic (obesity inducing) environment we now have in the United States today. If you make the same drive today, almost every exit is surrounded by fast-food restaurants. If you are just a little bit hungry, you are enticed to stop and eat. And of course the food isn't the best.

College also required some walking, but less than what I did in high school. The first 2 years in college, when I lived on campus, I walked about 20 minutes from my dorm to the classroom buildings. And then in the afternoon I walked back. When an exam was given that involved math, I needed to use a slide rule to perform calculations because hand calculators were not available yet (I bought my first calculator during my senior year in college—a basic model from Texas Instruments with nothing more than addition, subtraction, multiplication, and division functions, and it cost about $100).

After college I went to graduate school at the University of Wisconsin. Madison, Wisconsin, must be the greatest place in the Universe to go to college or graduate school. Housing costs are low, the campus is beautiful and large, and the city of Madison is the coolest place in the United States. Also, it is literally "Bike City, USA!" And most of the 6 years I lived in Madison I mainly maneuvered around the city by bicycle. The summers were hot and perfect for riding around town. I remember one summer I was on three separate softball teams and I was always running out of the lab to catch a game. The downside was that the winters were excruciatingly cold and a little bit less comfortable to ride your bike. After several years I set the temperature cut off for riding my bike at 20 degrees Fahrenheit—not really because of the cold, but because the ice patches were too dangerous at that temperature or below.

My first Thanksgiving in Madison was interesting. One of my roommates was given a large turkey by the company she worked for. We were all standing in the kitchen and the discussion was, "What should we do with the turkey?" Not one of my roommates knew how to cook a turkey. I piped up and said, "I know how to cook a turkey, and I know how to make most of the side dishes, so I'll cook Thanksgiving dinner. And I did! As I explained in the previous chapter, I helped my mother make dinner when I was young. It is a skill that has helped me at college, at graduate school, while backpacking around the country, and it has also helped me in my career as a scientist. Cooking and performing laboratory work are very similar.

After 5 years in graduate school in Madison, when it came time to write my Ph.D. thesis, I needed to use a pencil to write out the chapters in long hand in the department library during the day, and then at night, I struggled typing my thesis on a typewriter. The Apple IIe was just becoming popular in the early 1980s (a graph on computer availability will be presented in a later chapter). I started writing my thesis on February 15, 1982, and defended my thesis in early December of that same year.

Conclusions

The conclusions from the above remembrances of the 1960s and the 1970s are that before the establishment of today's obesogenic environment, it was necessary to perform energy intensive physical activities in order to carry out everyday life activities. Even the process of making dinner in the home required work that helped burn kilocalories in the preparation of the family meal. Today, even in some cases if you still need to perform physical activities in the daily routine, it is easy to stop and consume a fast-food meal and obtain 1,000 kcal in under 10 minutes. This was not an option in the 1960s. Why the pre-1970s was less obesogenic than today revolved around the sum of everyday activities (often very small ones) that required energy expenditure, and the fact that it was not possible to quickly stop and eat a high kilocalories, fast-food meal. Also, super gigantic food stores were not the norm. Most people bought their food in small grocery stores or just slightly larger supermarkets, or in specialty shops such as a butcher for meat or a bakery for bread.

One purpose of this book is to show all the ways we have changed our lives that have made it more difficult to maintain a body weight that was the norm in the early portions of the 1900s. Showing the complexities involved in these changes will prevent us from swallowing misleading statements promulgated by "Internet nutrition experts" who want us to buy their books. Also, we will learn to maneuver around products developed by major food companies, who want us to continue to eat their kilocalorie-dense snacks and foods. The more they sell, the more money they make for their shareholders. The fact that the health of Americans are thrown to the wayside apparently makes little difference to them.

Food–In and Out of the Home

We just caught a look at how life was in the 1950s and 60s. The dynamics of eating changed in many ways in the second half of the 1900s. When I was a child we ate more than 95% (probably more) of our meals at home. Only occasionally did my family go out to eat, and every so often, I ate with my mother in a department store cafeteria or at the Automat. Why this dynamic changed is a wide ranging social question that is difficult to answer. Certainly, the rise in the fast-food industry was part of it. Also the changes in family roles and economics were involved. If I remember correctly and honestly, even though my Mom was a great cook, eating at home all the time was kind of boring. Increasing choice alone had an impact. One thing is for sure, the current foodscape is not going away without a major change in the way food is distributed and sold.

What Other Changes in Food Patterns Were Taking Place in the U.S. in the 1900s

I previously discussed the changes in the availability and usage of food commodities over the past 100 years or so. The main findings are summarized here:

a) The intake of grain (largely whole grains) decreased during the first 50 years of the 1900s, and then around 1970, intake of grain started to increase again (but mostly due to refined grains—especially wheat and corn flour). The intake of dietary fiber also decreased during the 1900s.

b) The intake of fat was the most important macronutrient contribution to the increase in Calories consumed during the period 1970 to 2004 and beyond. Some new fat products led the steady increase in fat intake, including shortening made from hydrogenated vegetable oils, soy oil, and chicken (chickens raised in the second half of the 1900s contained much more fat and lower omega-3 fatty acids than chickens grown earlier on small farms under free range conditions).[1]

c) Quite surprisingly, the intake of <u>total</u> added sweeteners stayed fairly consistent during the 1900s, but there was the introduction of a new sweetener—high-fructose corn syrup.

What Is the Current American Home with Young Children Like? And How Can It Be Transformed Into a Healthy Obesity-Resistant Home?

These questions were asked by Dr. Carol Byrd-Bredbenner of the Department of Nutritional Sciences at Rutgers University. She is the Principal Investigator and leads a research project called "HomeStyles."

The HomeStyles Research Project is designed to look at the modern day home environment of families, and to determine which family habits and practices lead to healthy nutrition and lifestyles in order to raise "healthier families." The HomeStyles research project also investigates the opposite—which practices lead to a less healthy family environment that may provide fertile ground for the onset and continuance of obesity.

As discussed in an article by Dr. Byrd-Bredbenner and her research team[2]: "To date, obesity interventions focused on prevention of weight gain in children under 5 years of age have shown limited effectiveness in reducing or limiting weight gain [9]. A systematic review of obesity prevention interventions among preschool children suggest the failure to show an intervention effect may be partly due to the lack of focus on social and environmental factors within which diet and physical activity behaviors are enacted [10]."

The HomeStyles study is in its early stages and is currently collecting and analyzing baseline data from control homes (those that have been initially enrolled). Parents of 489 preschool children completed a cross-sectional online survey for the

---

[1] Wang Y, Lehane C, Ghebremeskel K, Crawford MA (2010). Modern organic and broiler chickens sold for human consumption provide more energy from fat than protein. *Public Health Nutrition* 13(3): 400–408.http://journals.cambridge.org/action/displayAbstract?fromPage=online&aid=7190300&fileId=S1368980009991157

[2] Quick V, Martin-Biggers J, Povis GA, Hongu N, Worobey J, Byrd-Bredbenner C (2017). A socio-ecological examination of weight-related characteristics of the home environment and lifestyles of households with young children. *Nutrients* 2017 Jun 14;9(6). pii: E604. doi: 10.3390/nu9060604. https://www.ncbi.nlm.nih.gov/pubmed/?term=PMID%3A+++++28613270

purpose of collecting baseline information about the families enrolled in the HomeStyles program.

One of the goals of the study is to model home life so that activities that are obesogenic can be altered to reduce the obesity rate in a wide variety of homes. The study is wide reaching, and it investigates the current complex environment of the American home. The families recruited had younger children between 2 and less than 6 years old. The families were recruited from two states in the U.S.—New Jersey and Arizona.

The main areas of investigation of the HomeStyles research project are:

1. General Family Background—The general demographics of the family members and their environment.
2. Home security/environment—Personal organization, control of stress, household chaos, emotional environment at family mealtime, and levels of family conflict.
3. Food security—Which families had adequate income to provide nutritious food.
4. Diet and meals—Meal-planning behaviors, skill in preparing family meals, specific dietary intakes (e.g., fruits and vegetables, milk, sugar-sweetened beverages, fat), typical availability of fruit/vegetable juice, amount of salty/fatty snacks, sugar-sweetened beverages in the home.
5. Eating outside the Home—The general circumstance and frequency of eating family meals in various locations (e.g., in the car or in a restaurant).
6. Access to technology—Home media environment (i.e., number and types of media digital devices in the home and in child's bedroom); amount of daily screen time children were allowed.
7. Exercise in the home and yard—The amount of space and devices available for physical activity inside the home and immediately near by the home (yard).
8. Exercise outside the home—Parent and child actively playing together; parents being role models by exercising; parental encouragement of children's physical activity; importance and value parents placed on physical activity; availability of parks and playgrounds to play in neighborhood, along with perceived neighborhood safety and frequency of outdoor active play.
9. Sleep—Investigated all aspects, including sleep duration of parents and children.

What are the results of the HomeStyles program so far (as of December 2017)? Since the enrolled families had just been recently recruited, the results so far are baseline information about the group.

1. Parents and children in these young families were generally healthy despite homes that were fairly disorganized, and where parents were under stress.

2. Daily intakes of 100% fruit/vegetable juice and milk were low at slightly more than half a serving daily, and they were lower than the intake of sugar-sweetened beverages daily intake.

3. Fat intake was slightly more than one-third of total daily calories.

4. Physical activity was low, and screen time (sedentary) was extremely high (~6 hours/day). The last two observations are very common findings these days!

5. Inside active play was only moderate. Play immediately outside in the neighborhood was more active.

6. Frequent family meals were a plus. Family meals at the dining table were eaten nearly twice per day.

7. Parents were able to promote physical activity-related childhood obesity protective practices.

8. The HomeStyles study did, indeed, identify lifestyle practices and home environment characteristics that health educators could target to help parents promote optimal child development and lower childhood obesity.

9. In general the surveyed households were chaotic but with low family conflict.

10. Parents agreed that family meals provided a positive emotional environment. Parents agreed that active planning for healthy meals was important and that physical activity led to positive outcomes. Half the time TV was watched during family meals or snacking. But in general there was poor ability to model or institute healthy practices.

11. The parents averaged 7 hours of sleep per night while the preschoolers' average total sleep duration (naps and nighttime sleep) was almost 11 hours, but 28% got less than the recommended amount. Bedrooms (56%) had at least one digital device.

The overall conclusions from HomeStyles so far:

The current American home is disorganized (e.g., late for appointments, chores are put off, and meal times are not dependable), contains a high stress environment, and is chaotic (i.e., often resembling a noisy carnival).

Providing a healthy home environment would involve "obesity- protective behaviors (e.g., diet, physical activity, sleep, parent behavior modeling)" as well as "behavioral characteristics (e.g., parent organizational skills, need for cognition, stress, household organization)."

The biggest question I can see concerning the observations from the HomeStyles program is: Why is the current American home in need of so much help?

In my remembrances of my childhood and my family life in Brooklyn, the one main notable difference between my home life and those of today's modern family was the level of complexity and organization. In general, my home had one television in the living room, one parent (in my case—my mother) was home during the day and would keep the family organized and healthy. My mother would clean the house, organize belongings, perform small amounts of food shopping (my father did major grocery shopping on the weekends), make homemade nutritious meals, and in general keep track of anything and everything, including my whereabouts. We had a washer in the kitchen but no dryer. Clothes were hung out on a clothes line or put on a drying rack. All of these activities kept the family organized. In the bedrooms there were no televisions. In the room that I shared with my brother (from elementary school years to high school), we had a boom box type of record player and a radio. There were drawers, a desk, and beds—but nothing else. There were a minimum numbers of toys or other belongings in the bedrooms. My mother kept a "tight ship!"

In the summer there was no air conditioning, so it was more comfortable being outside than staying indoors. This included early evenings when most people sat on their stoops and discussed every subject imaginable. There were plenty of eyes to keep watch on the goings and comings of everyone—so safety was not a concern. Sometimes in the very hot weather, we would sleep outside in the backyard on cots with just white cotton sheets to cover us and protect us from mosquitoes.

Maybe our lives are just too complicated? Hopefully the HomeStyles research project will provide hard evidence of the reasons for our current obesogenic environment, and will provide reasonable solutions.

Let's Take a Deeper Look at What Changes in Food Consumption Occurred during the Period 1970 to Approximately 2008

The earlier chapters dealt with how the sources of foods changed and how newly conceived foods appeared in supermarkets. The following are figures and quotes taken from websites and publications of the Economic Research Service/USDA. Although the data are a little old, it gives a good snapshot of what was happening right after the Obesity Explosion. This group of scientists is responsible for tracking the trends in food consumption in the United States. Some of these data were presented earlier in this book, but the following are official graphs released by the Economic Research Service.

The next figure shows how the intake of poultry increased steadily during the Obesity Explosion while the intake of red meat declined. However, total meat consumption stayed level. Also note that intake of fish stayed constant throughout the period, but at an extremely low value.

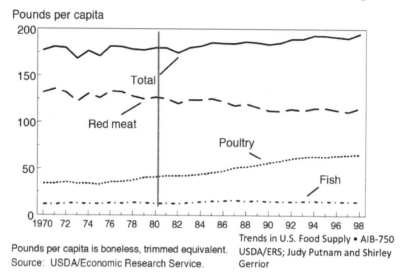

In 1998, total per capita meat consumption (196 pounds) was 19 pounds above the 1970 level--a new record high

Pounds per capita is boneless, trimmed equivalent.
Source: USDA/Economic Research Service.

Trends in U.S. Food Supply • AIB-750
USDA/ERS; Judy Putnam and Shirley Gerrior

The following figure shows one positive change made in the U.S. diet. The intake of whole milk decreased while the intake of reduced fat milk increased. Milk remains an important food for children in today's current home. In 1970, whole milk constituted about 83% of the total milk consumed. Whole milk now only amounts to 30% of the milk consumed. Reduced fat milk products are no doubt healthier for children and adults. Unfortunately, total per capita milk consumption dropped about 20% from 1970 to 1997.

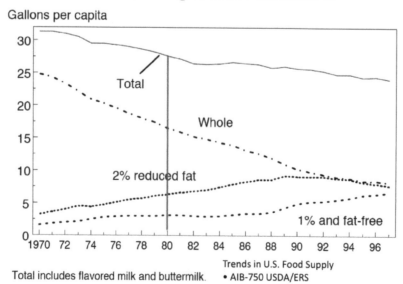

Americans are switching to lower-fat milks ...

Total includes flavored milk and buttermilk.

Trends in U.S. Food Supply
• AIB-750 USDA/ERS

However, since 1945, the intake of carbonated soft drinks (those containing sugar or other sweeteners) climbed steadily while total milk consumption decreased. By 1975, the per gallon consumption of each was about even. By 1992 the difference expanded to greater than 2 to 1, soft drinks to total milk consumed.

In 1945, Americans drank more than four times as much milk as carbonated soft drinks; in 1997, they downed nearly two and a half times more soda than milk.

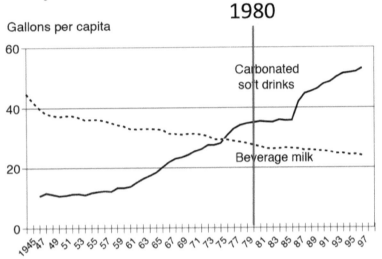

1947 is the earliest year for which data on soft drink consumption are available.

Per capita consumption of milk reached an all-time high in 1945 (data series dates from 1909).

... but cheese consumption continues to rise

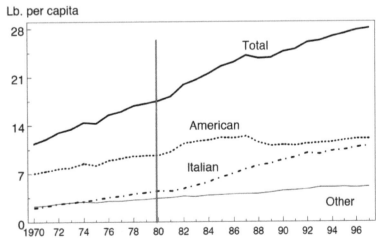

Natural equivalent of cheese and cheese products. Excludes full-skim American and cottage-type cheeses.

Trends in U.S. Food Supply • AIB-750 USDA/ERS; **Judy Putnam and Shirley Gerrior**

Source: USDA/Economic Research Service.

Cheese consumption increased steadily from 1970–1997. This probably more than compensated for the decrease in milk fat during the same period.

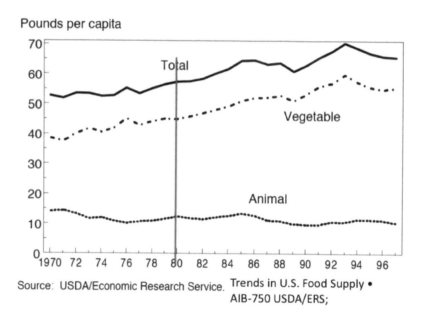

Vegetable-based products represent an increasing share of total added fats and oils consumption

Source: USDA/Economic Research Service. Trends in U.S. Food Supply • AIB-750 USDA/ERS;

The above data concerning the source of fats consumed by Americans agrees with the increases in shortening and soybean oil presented earlier. This presentation highlights that vegetable added fats contributed to the Obesity Explosion whereas animal-based added fats did not. This observation applies to the weight gain observed in Americans. This data has nothing to do with the relative health consequences of the fats, which have to be studied specifically for their effects on cardiovascular and overall health.

Food Consumed in the Home versus Food Consumed Away from the Home

In the chapter on growing up before obesity, I indicated that there were fewer places to eat food outside of the home in the 1950s and 1960s than there are today (2020), at least where I lived in Brooklyn. A major change in our economy has been the growth of the service food industry, especially the fast-food industry! In the next two figures from the Economic Research Service of the USDA, the Home versus Away food practices of Americans are explored over the time when obesity exploded.

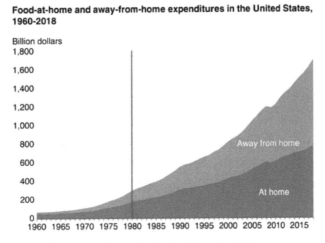

Food-at-home and away-from-home expenditures in the United States, 1960-2018

Source: USDA, Economic Research Service, Food Expenditure Series.

In the above figure the percent of the food budget spent for food prepared in the home started out in 1970 at about 75% of the food budget. It declined all through the period so that by 1996, the percentage spent for the home was down to 60%. In contrast, the percent of the budget spent for food outside the home increased steadily through the period—up to 40% by 1996. By 2009, the food spending reached 50.1% spent away from home. In 2018, the value increased to 54.4 percent of food expenditures were spent for food eaten away from the home.[3]

The following figure shows where the outside the home food sales are being made. Actually, the rise in eating at fast-food restaurants is responsible for a good deal of the increase in food being consumed outside the home. No surprise here!

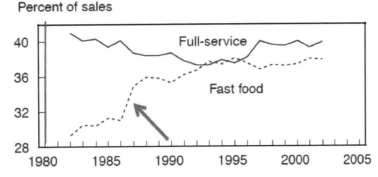

The away-from-home market by outlet type

Source: Food CPI, Prices, and Expenditures: Expenditure Tables. Economic Research Service.

Agricultural Report # 829   Economic Research Service/USDA

---

[3] Data from the USDA. See https://www.ers.usda.gov/data-products/ag-and-food-statistics-charting-the-essentials/food-prices-and-spending/

The Growth of the Largest Chain of Restaurants on a World Wide Basis

What about the growth of commercial outlets that allowed for greater and easier access to food outside the home over this same time period? The images below show the growth of a popular sandwich restaurant chain as reported by Venessa Wong and Steph Davidson of Bloomberg Businessweek (from August 26, 2013). I am presenting this data <u>only</u> to illustrate the tremendous growth in the availability of food outside the home over the past 40 years. It is amazing how this chain restaurant has spread throughout the world. **In no way am I associating the growth of this restaurant chain with the obesity crisis in the U.S.! This chain is one of many food restaurant chains that have spread over the U.S. and the world. This information demonstrates how food companies have embraced the global economy.**

Global Spread of Subway Restaurants, the largest chain in the world

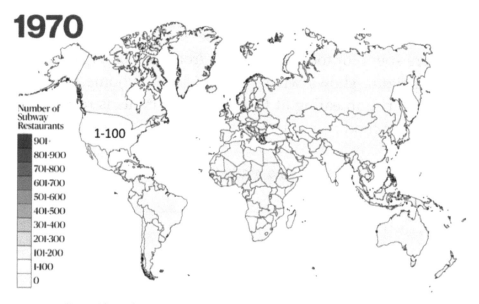

From Bloomberg Businessweek, by Venessa Wong and Steph Davidson, August 26, 2013

Global Spread of Subway Restaurants, the largest chain in the world

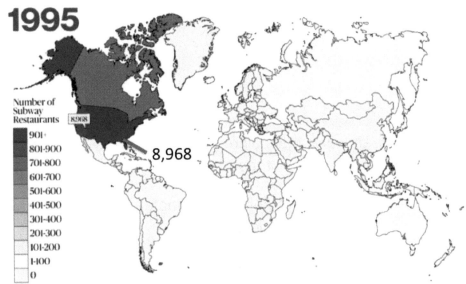

From Bloomberg Businessweek, by Venessa Wong and Steph Davidson, August 26, 2013

Global Spread of Subway Restaurants, the largest chain in the world

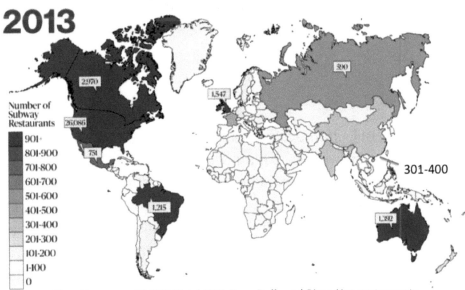

Also, there are 40,000 Total KFC, Taco Bell, and Pizza Hut restaurants world-wide! Including 14,000 outside the US!

Summary

The following general observations were made in this chapter concerning food intake in American homes.

Intakes of total meat were maintained, but red meat decreased and the consumption of chicken steady increased as percentage of sales.

Total fat intake was increased, largely due to increases in the consumption of shortening, soy oil, and fat laden chicken.

Overall, milk consumption was decreased.

Cheese consumption was increased. Carbonated beverage intake increased.

Fast-food restaurants not only proliferated in the U.S., but they also spread around the world.

50% of the food budget is now spent in eating outside the home.

Conclusions

The dynamics of family home life changed dramatically during the Obesity Explosion. More on this will be explored in coming chapters. Total kilocalorie intake per day increased and both fat (to a larger extent) and carbohydrate intake (due to the intake of refined flours and not sweeteners) increased over this period of time, too. The blame game when it comes to macronutrients in the diet has been used by hundreds of the so-called "media nutrition experts" to write books that are purchased by unsuspecting consumers. Unfortunately, this blame game is nothing more than a giant red herring.

In the next chapter, we will look at another great change (The Rise of Digital Media), that occurred in society after the 1970s, that contributed to Obesity Explosion in the U.S.

The Role of Digital Media in the Obesity Explosion

Anyone who grew up in the 1950s and 1960s like I did could not have envisioned all the technological advancements (although Arthur C. Clarke envisioned a great many of them even earlier!)[1] that occurred in the late 1900s and now into the 2000s. When I was a young, no kid I knew would stay inside on a nice day, even if it was cold. Essentially there was nothing to do inside the home of the day. The house or apartment was where your mother ruled and played hostess when her friends visited. Times were certainly different, and we are influenced by what we did when we were young. When I teach, it astounds me that the one comment I make that my students find especially hard to believe is that I have not played a video or computer game since the original Pong and Pac-Man—sometime in the early 1980s? Computer games just do not interest me. But far more amazing than the capabilities of today's digital devices are their effects on the amount of time Americans engage in movement. Sitting for 8 to 10 hours at a time is not uncommon in the current digital world. This chapter explores the effects of the digital revolution on movement and the Obesity Explosion!

In previous chapters, I documented changes that occurred in available commodities and food consumption in the period after 1970. If that was all that occurred, it is possible that the energy regulation system in most individuals would have been able to withstand the powerful forces that they faced in the form of ubiquitous super palatable foods.

---

[1] Clarke AC (1999). *Greetings, Carbon-Based Bipeds: Collected Essays, 1934–1998.* (Edited by Ian T. Macauley). New York: St. Martin's Press (Given to me by my son Patrick, another forward thinker).

But in addition to the major changes that occurred, including the availability of myriad new foods and the explosion in fast-food restaurants in every region of the country, another major explosion was taking place across the landscape of America.

At the exact same time that there were major changes in food supply and consumption, there also occurred an explosion in the ways Americans accessed media—all due to the advances made in transistor-based technologies.

Before discussing the assault of digital devices on the lives of Americans, it would be interesting to investigate the viewpoint that Steve Jobs, a co-founder of Apple Computer, expressed concerning allowing his children to use digital devices in their home. Nick Bilton, a technology reporter for the *New York Times*, asked Mr. Jobs in 2010, "So, your kids must love the iPad?" Mr. Jobs answered, "They haven't used it. We limit how much technology our kids use at home." Mr. Bilton later asked Walter Isaacson, who knew Steve Jobs well, what was the Jobs' home like? Mr. Isaacson answered, "Every evening Steve made a point of having dinner at the big long table in their kitchen, discussing books and history and a variety of things. . . No one ever pulled out an iPad or computer. The kids did not seem addicted at all to devices."[2]

Unfortunately, many homes in the U.S. were not so insulated from the effects of digital devices as the home of Steve Jobs. The graph below shows the history of television (TV) sets and peripherals over the first 75 years of TV.[3] By around 1960, over 90% of households owned a black and white TV. By 1980, over 80% of households contained a color TV, and about 50% of households held more than one TV. But starting at around 1980, additional changes occurred in American households concerning television viewing. At around 1980, the percent of houses wired with cable television was only 20%, but by the year 2000, this percent had increased to 70%. Slightly after 1980, remote controls and video cassette recorders (VCRs) started to appear in homes. By 1990, 70% to 80% of households already contained remote controls and VCRs. In a 10-year period starting in 1980, the way Americans watched and utilized televisions and related equipment became much more sophisticated and diverse. VCRs allowed Americans to watch movies that were previously unavailable except during short intervals of time. The appearance of the VCR spawned a new cottage industry—the neighborhood video cassette store (now extinct due to online streaming).

The VCR data is especially interesting and relevant to me because one of my favorite stories from when my son (born in 1988) was small was that he developed an apparent English accent because he had watched the film, *Mary Poppins*, so many

---

[2] Nick Bilton, *New York Times*, September 10, 2014.

[3] Data from a table found on: http://www.tvhistory.tv/facts-stats.htm This site contains statistics on early TV programs, TV manufacturers, and television history in general. The data was graphed by the author.

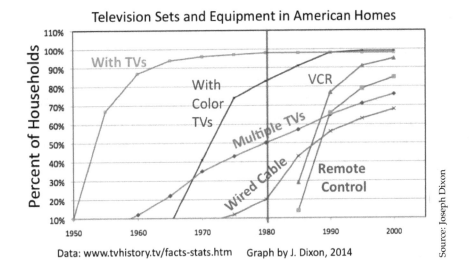

Television Sets and Equipment in American Homes

Data: www.tvhistory.tv/facts-stats.htm   Graph by J. Dixon, 2014

Source: Joseph Dixon

times. He also watched TV, but he especially liked to watch "Disney" movies that were becoming widely available on video cassette. The data on wired cable television shows that households began to receive many more stations than the locally available broadcast networks provided. The VCR and cable data accentuate the concept that the role of television in the home included much more than just watching network broadcast programming. TV evolved into a total entertainment center. MTV (originally Music Television) went on the air in August 1981 and at first just played music videos. Viewing sporting events became much easier as sports only programming channels appeared. For example, ESPN was launched in September 1979 and steadily increased in popularity. Since the birth of ESPN, sports only networks have proliferated on cable television, such that ESPN's popularity has decreased recently when competing sports stations chipped away at its viewership. By 2007 the average American home received 119 channels, including 17 broadcast TV stations (Nielsen).[4]

There is quite a substantial literature concerning the effects of watching television on the activity levels of children and adults. I will refer to some of these studies below and in a later chapter. But just observing how television and all of its connecting media suddenly expanded in complexity leads to the straightforward hypothesis that physical activity was strongly curtailed by all the extra time spent watching various forms of media in the home.

If this was all that happened during this time period, Americans may have been able to adapt to the lower activity levels that accompanied the explosion in television viewing. But another very large technological advance also occurred at this time that would go on to have great effects on both home life and work performed in the office.

---

[4] Data is from: www.nielsen.com/us/en/press-room/2008/average_u_s_home.html

Computers in Our Lives

When I was writing my Ph.D. thesis in 1982, I would write in the library using paper and pencil during the day, and later at night, when it was quiet in the lab, I would type what I had written during the day using a typewriter. A colleague from my lab was also writing his Ph.D. thesis at the same time. However, he was using a desktop computer that had just become available in Madison, Wisconsin. The computer he was using was the Apple IIe. I was slightly jealous of him, but there was nothing I could do, because there were no other similar computers in our entire building. Interestingly, we both completed our writing in late fall 1982. Therefore, I remember quite vividly when desktop computers became routinely available for practical writing purposes.

In the table below the production and shipping of desktop computers is shown from their introduction in the 1970s to the year 2011.

Computers, Smartphones, and Tablet Sales, 1975-2010

	Computers	Smartphones	Tablets
		(Millions of units per year)	
1975	very low		
1980	0.5		
1985	5		
1990	20		
1995	60		
2000	150	0	
2005	220	70	0
2010	360	360	30

Values are total units shipped for the year across all manufacturers. Data was compiled from several websites including https://arstechnica.com (Values reported by Jeremy Reimer on August 14, 2012). Red line denotes Obesity Explosion.

The table shows in 1975 very small amounts of personal computers were shipped. By 1980 the number was up to a half a million per year. And by 1995, around 60 million computers were being shipped per year. Again I have a personal recollection of this time as my 5-year-old daughter (born in 1991) had mastered all of the computer game programs that were available for the Macintosh computer in our local library. We would go to the library and I would read or do work sitting in a place where I could observe her in the computer room. The library owned 15 different programs for children and my daughter would sit in front of the computer for several hours without lifting her head. Before my eyes I was seeing the amazing mesmerizing capabilities of the desktop computer. Therefore, by approximately 1995, there were fairly sophisticated games that could be played by children for hours and hours. I was there and personally observed this!

The figure below breaks up the different kinds of computers that were made during this period. The data plotted in this graph shows the introduction of computers during the first years of the personal computer.

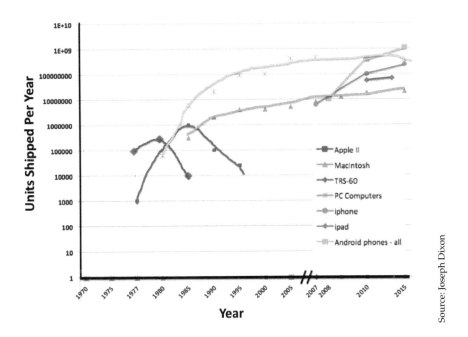

Source: Joseph Dixon

The Effects of Digital Devices and Media on Physical Activity and Health

The table below shows the times that were spent watching television versus surfing the internet by computer in the English adult population in 2006. It is suitable to illustrate this data for this time because it resided within the Obesity Explosion period. The data, collected by IBM,[5] show that respondents used the Internet approximately as many hours as they watched television. Seventy-three percent of the respondents cruised the internet 2 or more hours/day whereas 63% of the same group watched television 2 or more hours per day. The researchers suggested that part of the reason for this observation were the extra hours that were used to surf the internet during personal time at work. The upshot of this study was that adults could spend the same number of hours, or more, surfing the Internet as watching TV.

---

[5] Figures are from: http://www.nmk.co.uk/article/2006/8/30/switching-channels

Comparison of Television versus Internet Usage in Adults in England

	Daily Television	Daily Internet Usage (Home and Work)
Under 1 hour	8%	4%
1 to 2 hours	28%	24%
2 to 4 hours	39%	38%
4 to 6 hours	17%	18%
Over 6 hours	7%	17%

Values are are from a study by IBM and posted on:
http://www.nmk.co.uk/article/2006/8/30/switching-channels.
Retrieved on January 20, 2012.

There are many studies that describe the effects of increasing the use of electronic media on physical activity and health. The above figures show that the influx of all the possible ways to spend time using electronic media led to a convergence of effects such that we have been transformed into a largely sedentary society.

Tremblay et al. performed a systematic analysis of 232 studies with a total enrollment of almost one million children.[6]

The authors concluded,

"Qualitative analysis of all studies revealed a dose-response relation between increased sedentary behaviour and unfavourable health outcomes. Watching TV for more than 2 hours/day was associated with unfavourable body composition, decreased fitness, lowered scores for self-esteem and pro-social behaviour and decreased academic achievement."

In the same article the authors related that Intervention studies showed that many of the above negative effects were reversed when children spent less than 2 hours/day viewing television.

Increased television availability and viewing not only decreased daily physical activity, but it also affected sleep in children. The presence of television sets in

---

[6] Tremblay MS, LeBlanc AG, Kho ME, Saunders TJ, Larouche R, Colley RC, Goldfield G, Gorber SC. (2011) Systematic review of sedentary behaviour and health indicators in school-aged children and youth. *International Journal of Behavioral Nutrition and Physical Activity* 8: 98 Online open access: http://www.ijbnpa.org/content/8/1/98

the bedrooms of children was observed to significantly shorten their nightly sleep time.[7]

Convergence of Use of Digital Media on Sedentary Behavior in the U.S.

The CDC collects yearly data concerning the level of physical activity (and its opposite, inactivity) throughout the United States. The CDC data are remarkable, and one can easily go to the CDC website in order to view PowerPoint slides that show the year-by-year increases in inactivity, as well as the increases in the obesity rates and the increases in the number of diagnosed cases of type 2 diabetes in the U.S.[8] Every semester I have students in my class explore these CDC statistics.

I was amazed how the maps for the different parameters had similar distributions showing the areas of high incidence of inactivity and disease throughout the U.S. In the next figure, I placed the distribution maps for inactivity, obesity, and diabetes on the same slide. The similar distributions are eye opening!

In the following slide, seven regions with extremely high inactivity are demarcated:

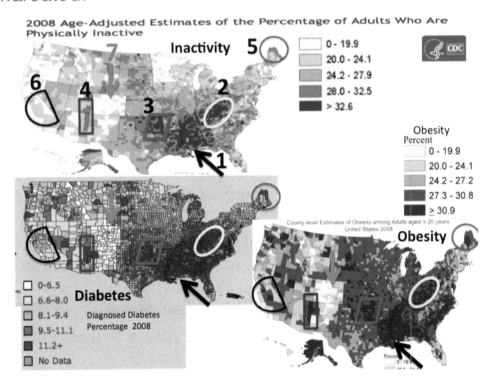

---

[7] Cespedes EM, Gillman MW, Kleinman K, Rifas-Shiman SL, Redline S, Taveras EM. (2014) Television Viewing, Bedroom Television, and Sleep Duration From Infancy to Mid-Childhood. Pediatrics 133: e1163–e1171. http://pediatrics.aappublications.org/content/133/5/e1163.full.html

[8] Website: http://www.CDC.gov/diabetes

Closeup of Inactivity Map:

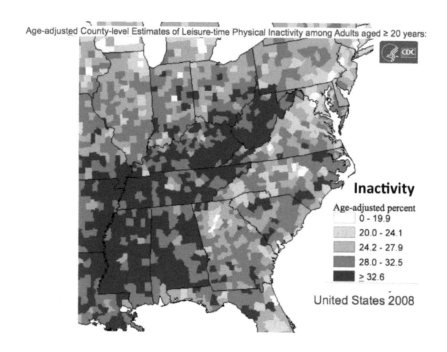

The seven highly inactive areas indicated on the map are summarized here:

1. The states of Louisiana, Mississippi, Alabama, Tennessee, Kentucky, and West Virginia have high rates of inactivity, obesity, and type 2 diabetes.

2. Eastern Kentucky and most of West Virginia have extremely high rates of inactivity and obesity (see map closeup).

3. Eastern Oklahoma has a dense area of inactivity, obesity, and diabetes.

4. There is a narrow strip in western Arizona and southern Utah that represents the location of various Native American tribes that have high rates of inactivity, obesity, and diabetes.

5. Northern Maine has a region of overlapping high rates of inactivity, obesity, and diabetes.

6. There is an elongated region of central California that represents the central valley that has overlapping high rates of inactivity, obesity, and diabetes. There is much less inactivity (i.e., more activity) along the coast of California.

7. The one bright spot in the U.S. is Colorado, where there are light areas for all the parameters, thus there are relatively lower rates of inactivity, obesity, and diabetes in Colorado compared to all other regions of the U.S.

The maps (from 2008) depict extremely strong data that point convincingly to the role of inactivity in the obesity epidemic. Why are these areas especially prone to inactivity and obesity? The answers are complex and they differ from state to state and area to area. Obesity is also the result of other factors such as healthy food deserts and an obesogenic built environment. Some of the possible nonnutrition reasons for the high rates of low inactivity are listed below:

1. High inactivity in areas of the Deep South may be due to high summer temperatures and humidity, forcing people to stay indoors in air conditioning during these months.
2. High summer temperatures and humidity may also be the reason for high inactivity in Eastern Oklahoma and Eastern Kentucky and most of West Virginia, too.
3. Northern Maine may have the opposite situation where the very long, cold winters keep people inside.
4. The narrow strip in eastern Arizona is populated by native American tribes who live on reservations that are located in areas with extremely high summer temperatures. In addition, it is well known that Native Americans have "thrifty" metabolism that leave them susceptible to obesity when a "western type diet" is consumed.[9]
5. The State of Colorado is a region of higher relative recreational activity and, therefore, is somewhat resistant to the increase in obesity found in other areas of the U.S.

Will the Digital Revolution End Up Reversing the Obesity Explosion?

Many of my students read this chapter for my 2017 Spring and Fall Nutrition and Health classes. And many of them pointed out that they thought digital devices, especially the smart phone, would eventually help solve the Obesity Explosion in the future. I had not even considered this because I was not up on the current programs or Apps that have been designed to help people become healthier. After this experience, as an assignment, I give students an essay that addresses the future use of the start phone as a device that enhances health rather than causing people to spend even more time being inactive.

Conclusions

It is true that all of the data presented in this chapter consist of associations—such is the nature of life. Not every aspect of life can be measured in a random controlled double blind study. But starting in the 1970s and 1980s, very large

---

[9] Carey MC, Paigen B. (2020) Epidemiology of the American Indians' burden and its likely genetic origins. *Hepatology* 36(4 Pt 1):781–91 https://pubmed.ncbi.nlm.nih.gov/12297824

eruptions occurred in our society that led a large percentage of individuals, especially children, to change habits such that our country went from a population that performed moderate physical activity to a population that was largely immovable and sedentary.

The unmistakable conclusion that can be extracted from all the data that were presented in this chapter is that a significant portion of the increase in obesity, starting in 1970, was the result of waves of advances in digital media and the adoption of these in every aspect of life. Of especial importance were the introductions of cable TV, VCRs, and the remote control device, which collectively led to more sophisticated media viewing. Then barely 15 years later, there was an infusion of desktop computers, such that by the year 2000, most households had both sophisticated television systems and easy to use desktop computers available for attention addiction. The introduction of each of these two major digital systems caused a powerful assault on the biology of humans, such that the energy regulation systems that were developed over millions of years of evolution were completely overloaded and outmoded within a short 30-year period. Thus, the Obesity Explosion that occurred around 1980 and that continues today.

The Contribution of Politics and Income Inequality to the Obesity Explosion

All throughout the 10,000-year history of agriculture, there were threads of social stratification where the leaders, administrators, and professional soldiers ate the most nutritious food; whereas the peasants, who worked long hours in the fields, made due with whatever crops that were not collected for taxes. This arrangement led to a healthier and stronger central authority, and a dutiful, weaker peasant population, who were constrained to work long days. This orderly arrangement still echoes in our current society where those in lower economic strata have less access to health care, nutritious food, and a healthy physical environment. One of the ramifications of all this is that those who suffer from income inequality have a higher rate of obesity. How ironic is that?

Wealthy countries have higher rates of obesity than poor countries, but within the wealthy United States, poorer counties have greater obesity rates than richer counties. This was made clear in the U.S. in the figure that placed the distribution maps for inactivity, obesity, and diabetes within the same image. The highest rates of obesity correlated with some of the poorer areas in the U.S.

Dr. James Levine wrote the following in a recent editorial concerning the role of poverty in the obesity crisis[1]: "Poverty is an ignored cause of obesity . . . Of the 220,256 articles written by scientists about obesity, <1% of manuscripts address poverty." "Similarly, at clinicaltrials.gov, less than 3% of the 6209 obesity trials, address issues of poverty."

---

[1] Levine JA (2015). Solving obesity without addressing poverty: Fat chance. *J Hepatol* 63: 1523–1524. http://www.journal-of-hepatology.eu/article/S0168-8278%2815%2900520-6/abstract

The following figure shows that income inequality has widened since 1980 in the United States and in some other Western countries.[2] As of 2014, around 20% of all income in the U.S. went to the top 1% of Income households. This redistribution of wealth was also observed, but to a lesser extent, in the United Kingdom and Canada. It is interesting to note that the current inequality level is similar to what it was in the 1920s before the great depression. The entire range of the effects of inequality, including income inequality, on the American democracy was examined by Nobel winning economist, Joseph E. Stiglitz, who has written that the United States has the greatest inequality of any Western country.[3]

Income Inequality Is Real in the U.S.

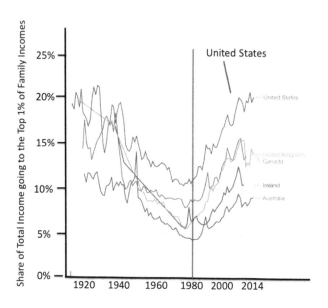

In his travels around the country, Dr. Stiglitz indicated that the question he is asked the most is, "When did we go astray?" He answered,[4,5]

> There is no easy answer to such a question, but clearly the election of President Ronald Reagan represented a turning point in the United States. Among the precipitating events were the beginning of the deregulation of the financial

---

[2] Share of Total Income going to the Top 1% since 1920. The data are from World Wealth and Income Database (2018). Income is before taxes and transfers. Licensed under CC-BY-Sa by Max Rosen. Retrieved from: 'https://ourworldindata.org/income-inequality' on 6-23-2020. Red line is the Obesity Explosion.

[3] Stiglitz JE (2013, paperback edition). *The Price of Inequality: How Today's Divided Society Endangers Our Future.* New York: W. W. Norton & Company.

[4] Stiglitz JE (2013, paperback edition). Ibid, page xxxi (preface to the Paperback Edition).

[5] President Ronald Reagan served as President from January 20, 1981–January 20, 1989.

sector and the reduction in the progressivity of the tax system. Deregulation led to the excessive financialization of the economy—to the point that before the 2008 crisis 40% of all corporate profits went to the financial sector. The path of deregulation upon which Reagan set the country was, unfortunately, followed by his successors. So was the policy of lowering the taxes at the top. First the top rates was lowered from 70% to 28% (under Reagan), and then (after Bill Clinton raised the top rate to 39.6% in 1993) they were lowered under George W. Bush to 35%... The result is that the top 400 income earners in the United States paid an average tax rate of just 19.9% in 2009.

The problem of income inequality is not just limited to effects on the poor and certain minority groups. Even middle aged non-Hispanic white men and women in the U.S. are not benefiting from advances in medicine and health care. The next figure shows "All-cause mortality" from 1990 to 2015 for the ages 45–54 years. The data were similar for other age groups below 60 years old for US white men and women (non-Hispanic). White Americans (non-Hispanic) have the highest median incomes in the U.S., but their mortality rate (Red Line—WNH) did not decrease like it did in the comparison countries. The conclusion from these observations is that even Americans (the middle class) who historically were in the upper 50% of incomes have not kept up in real income and are not benefiting from the current health care system in the U.S. Whether the lack of improvement in all-cause mortality is due to poor nutrition, sedentary life styles, or not having access to adequate medical care is not precisely known. The fact that over 40% of Americans are obese (Chapter 2)

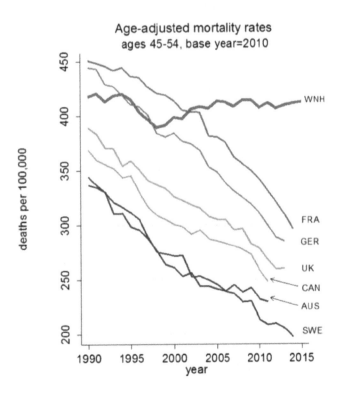

would lead to the hypothesis that all three are factors in continued high morbidity compare to other counties.[6]

Inequality, Children, and Food Insecurity

Many of the poorest Americans, especially children, experience food insecurity, which is essentially not knowing when or where the next nutritious meal will come from. Anderson (1990) stated that food insecurity occurs, "whenever the availability of nutritionally adequate and safe foods or the ability to acquire acceptable foods in socially acceptable ways is limited or uncertain."[7] It is the sad situation that poverty has become worse in the past 30 years—during the period of the Obesity Explosion.

In addition to some segments of our country becoming poorer, the United States has increased its incarceration rate 4-fold since the early 1970s.[8] The figure below shows how the total prisoner population held in state and federal prisons in the U.S. changed since 1960.[9] The increase in prison population was due to many reasons, but a large part was due to new sentencing laws that were part of the war on drugs and crime enacted in the late 1960s, and the Crime Bill enacted by President Bill Clinton later in 1994 (See Timeline in Chapter 4). Of course, the poor were the main recipients of the new sentencing laws and the number of families that lost fathers to incarceration skyrocketed. The ensuing increase in single-parent households increased the stress and anguish felt by both young mothers and children. Also, a larger percentage of the budget of state governments needed to be redirected to the cost of building and maintaining new prisons, and to the cost of keeping so many people behind bars. So less state funds were available for nutrition programs.

---

[6] Case A, Deaton A (2017). Mortality and morbidity in the 21st century (CONFERENCE VERSION). Prepared for the Brookings Panel on Economic Activity, March 23–24, 2017, p. 57.

[7] Anderson SA (1990). Core indicators of nutritional state for difficult-to-sample populations. *J Nutr* 120: 1559–1560. http://www.ncbi.nlm.nih.gov/pubmed/?term=Core+indicators+of+nutritional+state+for+difficult-to-sample+populations.

[8] Enns, Peter K. (2016) *Incarceration Nation: How the United States became the most punitive democracy in the world.* New York: Cambridge University Press, pages 3 and 4. See this book for comparisons of the U.S. with other western countries.

[9] Data are from Bureau of Justice Statistics, Key Statistics, Annual Probation Survey, Annual Parole, Survey, Annual Survey of Jails, Census of Jail Inmates, and National Prisoner Statistics Program, 1980–2016 (Date of version: 4/26/2018—See Excel Spreadsheet), on the Internet at www.bjs.gov (https://www.bjs.gov/index.cfm?ty=kfdetail&iid=487; visited 06-23-2020); and from: The Sentencing Project, https://www.sentencingproject.org/publications/trends-in-u-s-corrections/ (Fact Sheet: Trends in U.S. Corrections). Values are only for the population held in state and federal prisons and does not include those on probation or held in county jails. The vertical red line at 1980 denoted the Obesity Explosion.

Dr. Enns quoted Governor Arnold Schwarzenegger from his 2010 State of the State address as follows:

> The priorities have become out of whack over the years. I mean, think about it. Thirty years ago 10 percent of the general fund went to higher education and 3 percent went to prisons. Today, almost 11 percent goes to prisons and only 7.5 percent goes to higher education.[10]

Although the increase in the rate of U.S. incarceration and the increase in the rate of obesity in the U.S. are only tangential associations, their dramatic congruent nature is almost amazing.

U.S. State and Federal Prison Population, 1960 to 2016

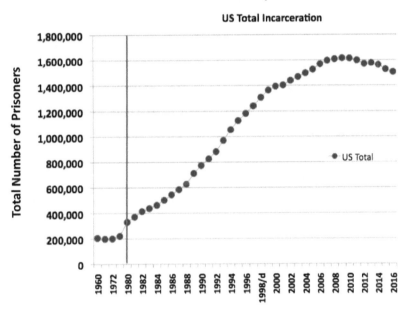

In a world full of ironies, a very sad yet interesting irony of the current Obesity Explosion is that poverty and food insecurity breeds obesity. It does this in several major ways.

1. Lack of funds to purchase nutritious foods and general food insecurity leads families to rely on relatively inexpensive, nutrient poor, energy dense foods, especially during the last week of the food stamp cycle.
2. Obese girls grow up to be obese mothers, who give birth to very large babies, who are at increased risk for becoming obese children, and the cycle of obesity is set up to continue.

---

[10] Enns PK (2016). Ibid, p. 6; Complete speech available at http://www.govspeech.org/pdf/19694d.pdf

3. Mothers and caregivers in poor neighborhoods keep their children safe by keeping them inside the house or apartment rather than allowing them to play outside where they may be exposed to violence as a result of drug abuse and gang activities. Since the children get bored staying inside watching television, mothers try to make their children content by buying them cheap, tasty, calorie dense snack foods.[11]

Let's address each of these in greater detail.

1. Lack of funds to purchase nutritious foods and general food insecurity…..

The USDA reported[12] that in households with children, 17% experienced food insecurity without hunger while less than 1% of their children experienced hunger. In households without children, 8% experienced food insecurity without hunger and 4% reported hunger. The low amounts of hunger in households with children is a result of the WIC program (The Special Supplemental Nutrition Program for Women, Infants, and Children [WIC]), which supplements other aid programs when families have children. School lunch programs also contribute to less hunger in children.

Dinour and colleagues carried out a review of studies of the effects of food insecurity on obesity in the literature published between 1996 and 2006.[13] In their article, the authors presented and discussed each study that they considered large enough and included well-described methods. They found a relationship between food insecurity and body weight in women, but not in men. This makes sense as men have more resources and spend a large amount of time out of the home.

Dinour and co-authors also found that there was no association between children in low-income households being overweight and food insecurity in the family. This last observation was also thought to be the result of the extra nutrition provided by the WIC program, and because mothers and caregivers often protect their children by giving them whatever nutritious food is available. However, an important wrinkle to this relationship occurred if the mothers in low-income households were obese, as will be discussed directly below.

---

[11] This last observation was also made by Dr. Debra Palmer Keenan, Ph.D., Associate Professor/Extension Specialist, during a lecture (Obesity, Income Inequality, and Obesity in the U.S.) she gave in my Class at Rutgers University: Obesity: Biology, Behavior, and Management (11:709:427:01), on November 15, 2017.

[12] USDA Economic Research Report # 11, 2004.

[13] Dinour LM, Bergen D, Yeh MC (2007). The food insecurity-obesity paradox: a review of the literature and the role food stamps may play. *J Am Diet Assoc* 107(11): 1952–1961. http://www.journals.elsevierhealth.com/periodicals/yjada/article/S0002-8223%2807%2901616-1/fulltext

2. Heavy girls grow up to be heavy mothers….

An explanation for continued increased obesity that applies specifically to infants and very young children is that, since we have been in the Obesity Explosion for at least 20 to 25 years, obese mothers are now giving birth to very large babies, who have a high probability of growing up obese. In fact, an article by Gorman's research group[14] indicated that, in the 28,000 children (2 to 5 years old) in the Massachusetts WIC program, the strongest association observed was that obesity in children was highly related to the birth weight of the infant.

The conclusions of the study by Gorman's group were:

"The results of this study point to a significant association between persistent household food insecurity without hunger, young children's weight status, and risk of childhood obesity. It is noteworthy, however, that the associations depend on maternal weight status. Given that results imply that specific groups of children are particularly vulnerable to adverse effects of household food insecurity, targeting these groups might be necessary."

But this study was informative in another straightforward way. And that was just the fact that there were, in the first place, 28,000 children in just one state who qualified for WIC aid. How can it be that in a highly developed, rich country, such as the U.S., there can be in one state 28,000 children who require nutrition assistance? And in a state like Massachusetts, which is one of our wealthiest states. If we multiply this number by 50, we come up with an extraordinary number of children in the United States who may require supplemental nutrition support.

So it appears that once obesity gets started, it can be easily be perpetuated when a cycle of generational obesity is set up to continue unless powerful interventions are put into place. As Dr. James Levine entitled his editorial, "Solving obesity without addressing poverty: Fat chance."[15]

3. Mothers or caregivers in poor neighborhoods prefer to keep their children safe by keeping them in the house or apartment….

The above was presented to my Obesity class in a lecture by Dr. Debra Palmer Keenan, an Associate Extension specialist and associate professor in the Department of Nutritional Sciences of Rutgers University.[16]

---

[14] Metallinos-Katsaras E, Must A, Gorman K (2012). A longitudinal study of food insecurity on obesity in preschool children. *J Acad Nutr Diet* 112(12): 1949–1958. http://www.andjrnl.org/article/S2212-2672%2812%2901514-6/fulltext

[15] Levine JA (2015). Solving obesity without addressing poverty: Fat chance. *J Hepatol* 63: 1523–1524. http://www.journal-of-hepatology.eu/article/S0168-8278%2815%2900520-6/abstract

[16] Discussed by Dr. Debra Palmer Keenan, Ph.D., Associate Professor/Extension Specialist, during a lecture (Obesity, Income Inequality, and Obesity in the U.S.) she gave in my Class at Rutgers University: Obesity: Biology, Behavior, and Management (11:709:427:01), on November 15, 2017.

Dr. Debra Palmer Keenan is an amazing health professional whose life's work is to help lower-income people have better lives and health through improved nutrition. But even more interesting is Dr. Palmer's own life story and educational path to become a faculty member at Rutgers University.

Dr. Debra Palmer Keenan grew up in the inner city of Cincinnati, Ohio. She realized that she needed to go to college in order to be successful and, as a single mother, she wished to give her son a better life and health insurance (he was asthmatic). Having always been strong in science and math in school, Dr. Palmer Keenan aimed high into the heavens and went for an Associate degree in aerospace engineering. Because during this time she needed food stamps to supplement the food in her home, Dr. Palmer Keenan interacted with other people who also required social services. Learning about nutrition programs rekindled her more terrestrial interests. After obtaining her undergraduate college engineering degree, Dr. Palmer Keenan taught physics and chemistry in high school in inner city schools. While teaching, Dr. Palmer Keenan realized that most inner city children had no idea how to successfully navigate modern society. This realization led Dr. Palmer Keenan to change her educational goals so that she could specifically help families in the inner city.

Dr. Palmer Keenan went on to earn two Master degrees, one in Education and the other in Nutrition. And later, she pursued a Ph.D. degree in Nutrition from Pennsylvania State University. Dr. Palmer Keenan traveled to the University of Minnesota for a first faculty position. It was in Minnesota where Dr. Palmer learned about government programs that were designed to help prevent hunger in the poor. One of them was Supplemental Nutrition Assistance Program—Education (SNAP-Ed, this was the education portion of the program formerly known as Food Stamp Nutrition Education [FSNE]). The other program was the Expanded Food and Nutrition Education Program (EFNEP). This program was specifically designed to help provide nutrition education to families with children.

After two years at the University of Minnesota, Dr. Palmer Keenan moved to New Jersey for a faculty position in Nutrition Sciences at Rutgers University. She set about using her knowledge to bring SNAP-Ed to New Jersey, and to make these government education programs efficient and helpful to the populations they were meant to serve. Having grown up in the inner city, and having received food stamps during the period she was attending college, Dr. Palmer Keenan was keenly aware of the special problems that face food-insecure people in urban areas. Dr. Palmer Keenan succeeded in bringing a more efficient and reliable food resource program to the State of New Jersey.

What Really Goes on in a Food-Insecure Home?

The cycles of food insecurity in families that Dr. Palmer studies in her research program at Rutgers University were more complicated than first imagined, and they widely differed among families and communities. But the following is a scenario that Dr. Palmer Keenan has observed in many families over and over again:

a) It is the underlying everyday life experiences in homes, and within families, that are important. People who are food insecure live under conditions and rules that are far removed from those who grow up with adequate incomes and with histories of belonging to mainstream America.

b) There is usually money for food during part of the month (½ to ¾ of the month), but there will be a period every month when there is little food in the apartment or house because of low paying hourly jobs and periodicity of assistance programs.

c) Caregivers shop in grocery stores that cater to lower-income neighborhoods. Cuts of meat, fruits and vegetables, and regular grocery items are usually of lower quality, but often are not much cheaper than those found in mega supermarkets that are in wealthier areas.

d) If the neighborhood is unsafe, then parents keep their children home, and therefore, children do not get exercise, fresh air, and sunlight. They also have less opportunities to play in parks and socialize with other children.

e) Because of long periods inside, parents will give their children the foods the children like or see advertised on television. These foods (often snack foods) are often unhealthy and obesogenic.

f) When life is extra stressful and the kids cannot go to activities because of lack of money or because of confrontations within the household, parents will keep children occupied with anyway they can and will feed them the cheapest food they can afford.

Dr. Palmer Keenan's experiences in New Jersey and her research articles point to the conclusion that successful and competent administrators need to understand the life experiences of the people in the communities they serve, and they need a broad educational background to know the biology and needs of humans. Being able to comprehend and navigate, like Dr. Palmer Keenan, the fairly complex laws of our government is also a major plus.

Please visit these websites for more information on Dr. Palmer Keenan's programs:
http://www.njsnap-ed.org
http://www.efnephelps.org
https://nutrition.rutgers.edu/faculty/debra-palmer.html

Income Inequality and Poverty Certainly Involves the Inside and Outside Physical Environments that People Live In

Anyone who travels around the metropolitan area that encompasses New Jersey, New York, and Connecticut already knows there has to be a better way to build a livable environment with safe and efficient transportation systems. The term, Physical-Built environment, a technical term defined as the bricks and mortar that compose the neighborhood environment where people (adults and children) live, eat, play, shop, work, and attend school. Therefore, the Physical-Built environment includes the neighborhood food environment, neighborhood parks and playgrounds, neighborhood walkability, neighborhood public transportation, and neighborhood safety. The Physical-Built environment, in most cases, cannot be altered unless the individual or family move to a new location.

In a review of studies on the effects of the Physical-Built environment on the development of obesity,[17] Booth and co-authors concluded that: "…….research presented in this review clearly demonstrate strong preliminary evidence of a relationship between built environment features and the prevalence of obesity. Lower SES (socioeconomic status-inserted by author) neighborhoods are a primary concern, as residents in these areas may have less access to recreational facilities or food stores with healthful, affordable options,……."

The impact of safe playgrounds on obesity in children was studied by Dr. Yanjong Jin of Rutgers University.[18] Dr. Jin used the 2007 National Survey of Children's Health (NSCH) to determine what effects the presence of a neighborhood park had on the obesity rate in children who live in different types of communities. Dr. Jin and her co-author found that the effects of a park/playground on childhood obesity was dependent upon many complex factors, including gender, age, race, household income level, neighborhood safety, and other neighborhood amenities. Of high importance was the safety of the neighborhood. As mentioned earlier,

---

[17] Booth KM, Pinkston MM, Poston WS (2005). Obesity and the built environment. *J Am Diet Assoc* 105: S110–S117. http://www.journals.elsevierhealth.com/periodicals/yjada/article/S0002-8223%2805%2900313-5/abstract

[18] Fan M, Jin Y (2013). Do neighborhood parks and playgrounds reduce childhood obesity? *Am J Agr Econ.* doi: 10.1093/ajae/aat047 First published online: August 6, 2013. http://ajae.oxfordjournals.org/content/early/2013/08/06/ajae.aat047.full

mothers will not allow their children to play in a park if they consider it an unsafe environment.

The Physical-Built Environment affects the health and upbringing of children differently based upon age and sex. The following groups of children received more protection from obesity by living near a safe neighborhood park:

1. The benefit was greater in girls than boys.
2. The benefit was greater in the 10 to 13 age group.
3. Non-Hispanic white youth benefited more than other groups of children in having a safe neighborhood park.
4. Children who lived in unsafe neighborhoods benefited more when the park was made especially safe using community patrols compared to control neighborhoods where the parks lacked enhanced security.

The take home message from Dr. Jin's research is that we need to consider the Physical-Built environment where people live when strategies to combat the Obesity Explosion are developed. However, if mothers are afraid to allow their children to play outside because of high levels of violence, it doesn't matter what Physical-Built environment is outside their homes. They will not let their children outside to play. When children are prisoners inside their home, the combination of inactivity coupled with eating high Calorie snack foods greatly increases the development of obesity.

Politics Fosters Income Inequality, Which Enhanced the Obesity Explosion

History has taught us that most examples of extreme hunger or starvation, either within single confined populations or across large areas of the globe are the result of fractional politics and war.[19] On the other hand, as described in this book, the Obesity Explosion is the result of many factors, including income inequality. Why is there inequality in the United States? According to Nobel Prize winning economist, Joseph Stiglitz, income inequality results from a system where a democracy, "based on one person one vote," is taken over by the 1 percent. Dr. Stiglitz goes on to describe how the 1%, essentially an oligarchy, slowly takes control of the political power in a country[20]:

> We described a process of disempowerment, disillusionment, and disenfranchisement that produces low voter turnout, a system in which

---

[19] Unklesbay NF (1992). *World Food and You*. Boca Raton, Florida: CRC Press (1st edition-paperback).

[20] Stiglitz JE (2013, paperback edition). *The Price of Inequality: How Today's Divided Society Endangers Our Future*. New York: W. W. Norton & Company, p. 183.

elected success requires heavy investments, and in which those with money have made political investments that have reaped large rewards—often greater than the returns on they reaped in their other investments.

No matter how income inequality became established in the U.S., the Obesity Explosion will not be contained until wealth is distributed more evenly. And with a more equitable distribution of wealth, access to better health care, education, and safer communities is required to turn the shock waves of the Obesity Explosion in the United States.

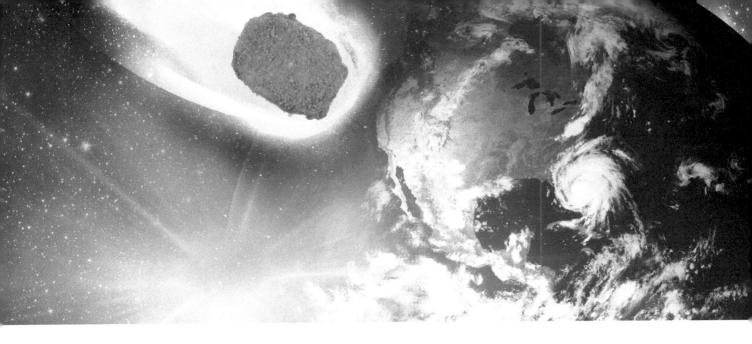

PART 4

How to Strive for Health

The Right Kind of Exercise is Important

We discovered that both digital media and income inequality influence activity on a daily basis. What is the role of exercise in the Obesity Explosion? This is an important question, and it is not as easy to answer as you might expect. After all, the increase in obesity over the past 50 years has correlated with the rise in the wearing of dedicated running and training shoes of all types! In fact, there is very serious debate among experts concerning what role exercise plays in the Obesity Explosion. Also, there are different types of exercise. The most important one for the maintenance of a healthy weight may surprise you!

The entire subject of the role of exercise in obesity was explored in the excellent article by James Hill, Holly Wyatt, John Peters.[1]

> There is considerable debate in the literature today about whether physical activity has any role whatsoever in the epidemic of obesity that has swept the globe since the 1980s. The timing of the secular rise in body weight fits so well with the expansion of food availability and marketing that it seems reasonable to assign significant blame to the food environment. Several arguments are made for this point of view. First, measures of leisure-time physical activity have not changed significantly over time. Second, measures of total energy expenditure have not declined over the time period during which obesity rates increased. This view, however, does not consider the necessary, but not sufficient, effect of the decline in physical activity that occurred in our society (and in those countries undergoing rapid urbanization and industrialization) during the first half of the 20th century.

---

[1] Hill JO, Wyatt HR, Peters JC (2012). Energy balance and obesity. *Circulation*. 126(1): 126–132. http://www.ncbi.nlm.nih.gov/pubmed/22753534

The last point made in the quote above is interesting because many devices (such as the clothes washer, the dish washer, and of course, the automobile) that directly have lowered our daily energy expenditure were invented during the first 50 years (maybe 60 years) of the 1900s. Therefore, the decline in energy expenditure was a forerunner of the Obesity Explosion that occurred around 1980.

Dr. Hill et al. go on to indicate that there are "...many studies showing that a high level of physical activity is associated with low weight gain over time and comparatively low levels of physical activity are associated with high weight gain over time." Church et al.[2] used data from the Occupational Safety and Health Administration and other government data to compare the energy requirements of jobs between 1960 and 2006. In 1960, 50% of the jobs required a fair level of physical activity. However, by 2006, less than 20% of the jobs had a similar level of activity. With so few Americans working in occupations that require physical activity, calculations of mean daily energy expenditure have fallen over this time. The research by Church et al. demonstrated that daily occupational energy expenditure decreased from a mean of 1,567 kcal/day in 1960 to 1,424 kcal/day in 2006. This small change in energy expenditure (just 143 kcal daily), when it happens every day over a long period of time (40 years or so), could, in fact, explain about half of the mean weight gain of Americans during the Obesity Explosion.[3]

Earlier I discussed Tremblay et al.'s systematic analysis of the role of activity in children and obesity in 232 studies with a total of almost one million children enrolled.[4] The authors stated, The authors concluded that watching TV for longer than 2 hours per day was associated with increased body weight and lower scores on tests that measure self-esteem, pro-social behavior, and academic achievement. The authors also indicated that the above negative changes could be reversed if children watched less than 2 hours of television per day.

I repeated the above observations because it is interesting that the 2-hour time point seems to be an important physiological marker for causing physiological changes in children. But what is just as interesting is that the 2- to 2.5-hour time point appears to be important in causing physiological changes in adults, too.

---

[2] Church TS, Thomas DM, Tudor-Locke C, Katzmarzyk PT, Earnest CP, Rodarte RQ, Martin CK, Blair SN, Bouchard C (2011). Trends over 5 decades in U.S. occupation-related physical activity and their associations with obesity. *PLoS One* 6(5): e19657. https://www.ncbi.nlm.nih.gov/pubmed/21647427

[3] Church T, Martin CK (2018). The obesity epidemic: A consequence of reduced energy expenditure and the uncoupling of energy intake? *obesity* 26, 14–16. https://www.ncbi.nlm.nih.gov/pubmed/29265774

[4] Tremblay MS, LeBlanc AG, Kho ME, Saunders TJ, Larouche R, Colley RC, Goldfield G, Gorber SC (2011). Systematic review of sedentary behaviour and health indicators in school-aged children and youth. *International Journal of Behavioral Nutrition and Physical Activity* 8: 98 Online open access: http://www.ijbnpa.org/content/8/1/98

In my nutrition and health class, students always ask about the role of structured exercise (performed in a gym, outside on a track, or at home on a treadmill, etc.) in treating obesity. I let them figure it out for themselves. I give them an assignment where they calculate their total daily energy expenditure and I have them list their favorite activities/exercise and the kilocalories (kcal) expended per hour during each activity. Then I have the students list their favorite snacks with the kilocalories each one has. The next step is to calculate how many hours he or she needs to exercise using their favorite activity/exercise in order to burn the Calories in their favorite snack. An example of this is given below for a woman or a man who is 64 kg (141 lb), who eats the red velvet cheesecake (1,250 cal/slice) (I admit, this is rather an extreme example) at a popular cheesecake restaurant. I also give more reasonable snacks.

Calories Expended Per Hour During Various Activities by a 141 pound (64 Kg):		Hours to work off Various Snacks:					
		Cheesecake 1250 Kcal		4 Oreos 212 Kcal		Banana 105 Kcal	
	Woman	Man						
	Kcal/Hour		Woman	Man	Woman	Man	Woman	Man
					Hours Required			
Biking	361	422	3.5	3.0	0.6	0.5	0.3	0.25
Running (10 min/mile)	589	688	2.1	1.8	0.36	0.3	0.18	0.15
Swimming Slow	346	405	3.6	3.1	0.6	0.51	0.3	0.26
Walking Brisk	244	285	5.1	4.4	0.9	0.74	0.43	0.37

Source: Joseph Dixon

The Calories per slice for the slice of the red velvet cheesecake was obtained from the www.myfitnesspal.com website. The activities listed and their energy expenditures were calculated from data provided on the National Academy of Sciences, Nutrition Research Council website.

It is extremely depressing to see that it requires 5.1 hours of brisk walking for a woman, or 4.4 hours of brisk walking for a man, to burn off the 1,250 cal in the slice of red velvet cheesecake that was probably eaten in under 10 minutes. Also quite amazing is the fact that the cheesecake contains 43 g of total fat! An acquaintance told me recently that he used to eat two slices of cheesecake every time he ate at the cheesecake restaurant. Needless to say, this was before his heart attack, and now he watches what he eats and swims regularly in the pool where I swim.

The reaction to this assignment has been consistent every year for the past 10 years: "I can't believe how long I need to exercise to burn off the kilocalories in my favorite snack!" It is just too easy in today's environment to eat excess kilocalories! The take home message from the class assignment is that structured exercise is not an effective nor efficient way to treat obesity, unless you have enormous amounts of time to spend in the gym (say 2 to 3 hours/day). I haven't met anybody who works full time with that kind of time yet! But an active lifestyle and a smart eating philosophy is critical to prevent a slow decline into the various stages of obesity.

What I teach in my class is that structured exercise is important and necessary for a healthy life for the following reasons:

Structured exercise:

1. Keeps coronary artery smooth muscle cells healthy so that they can dilate when your heart is called upon to pump extra blood—this will one day prevent you from having a heart attack;
2. Keeps ligaments and connective tissue strong and flexible so that you can avoid injuries;
3. Puts stress on your bones to keep them dense and strong;
4. Keeps skeletal muscles from dissolving away with age; and
5. Stimulates the release of endorphins, and later dopamine, in the brain.

An Amazing Fact about Walking as Exercise

It turns out that when you perform light to moderate exercise you are expending more fatty acids for energy than carbohydrate.[5] This is shown in the next figure (an adaptation of Figure 1 in the article; permission given by Dr. G. Brooks). Percent VO_2 max (maximal volume of oxygen consumed) corresponds to the effort exerted in exercise. At relatively low exertion levels, more fatty acids are used for muscle movement than glucose molecules. As exertion is increased, the substrates switch and glucose is used more than fatty acids. During very high-intensity exercise (90% to 100% VO_2 max), your muscles are primarily burning glucose. Therefore, low-intensity exercise should burn off more fat than glucose.

What about Strenuous Exercise?

Strenuous exercise is very good for many aspects of health. I always tell my students to exercise intensely 3–4 times/week to keep coronary artery smooth muscle cells and heart muscle cardiomyocytes healthy. The coronary artery smooth muscle cells are shown in the next figure. These cells are located between the internal elastic lamina and the artery connective tissue and are designated on

---

[5] Brooks GA, Mercier J (1994). Balance of carbohydrate and lipid utilization during exercise: the "crossover" concept. *J Appl Physiol* 76(6): 2253–2261. https://www.ncbi.nlm.nih.gov/pubmed/7928844

Brooks GA, Mercier J. J Appl Physiol 76(6): 2253-2261, 1994

the figure with a blue arrow. Although morphologically different, the coronary artery smooth muscle cells are like other muscle cells in that they need to be kept in good shape so that they react to different circumstances. They can relax to provide a wider diameter when called upon to deliver more oxygen to the heart. When less blood flow is needed in the heart and more is needed in other places like the intestine, the coronary artery smooth muscle cells will contract. Strenuous exercise will keep the coronary artery smooth muscle cells in good shape.

Strenuous Exercise Keeps Coronary Artery Smooth Muscle Cells in Good Shape

The coronary artery smooth muscle cells are similar to other muscle cells in that you have to use them or lose them. One of the reasons that diabetics die of CHD at rates four times higher than nondiabetics is that their coronary artery smooth muscle cells become very sick and are unable to relax and thus dilate the artery when more blood flow is needed, as when there needs to be compensation for a partial blockage of a main conduit artery in another region of the heart.

How Else Does Exercise Maintain Weight and Health?

Postprandial lipemia (blood triglyceride levels after the consumption of a meal) is higher in obese individuals. Women have lower postprandial lipemia than men (another way they are protected) and also have less heart disease than men.

People who are obese tend to have lower overall muscle and mitochondrial fatty acid oxidation in muscle. This was not reversed after weight loss, but it was improved with exercise training![6]

Exercise is a good way to prevent weight gain but is not so powerful in weight loss. The reason is that 1 hour of exercise is only 250 to 700 kcal/hour based upon the type of exercise. One can eat 700 kcal very easily in a matter of minutes!

It is obvious that the most powerful strategy for an individual to maintain basic health would be to prevent obesity from happening, because once it occurs, the basic evolutionary mechanisms to keep extra energy within the body kick in, and then it is very difficult to lose weight and fat stores!

An Exercise that May Be More Important Than Structured Exercise

There is an exercise that is very important in helping us maintain a healthy body weight. Dr. James A. Levine of the Mayo Clinic has spent a good part of his career researching and promoting the role of Non-Exercise Activity Thermogenesis (NEAT) in influencing a person's body weight.

What is NEAT? NEAT is the energy we expend each day in everyday activities such as walking, standing, cleaning the house, taking public transportation to work, walking the dog, standing instead of sitting, taking the stairs, and playing with the kids.

---

[6] Thyfault JP, Kraus RM, Hickner RC, Howell AW, Wolfe RR, Dohm GL (2004). Impaired plasma fatty acid oxidation in extremely obese women. *Am J Physiol Endocrinol Metab* 287: E1076–E1081. http://ajpendo. physiology.org/content/287/6/E1076.long

NEAT is the term for Non-Exercise Activity Thermogenesis. Thermogenesis in this case is the body mobilizing energy to move muscles, which will also generates extra heat. NEAT is a useful concept because it represents the Calories we expend at most jobs (such as walking around a store or restaurant, or sitting at a work station and occasionally walking to retrieve something) and what we do the rest of the day at home (daily chores and everyday movement). Activities that can be classified as NEAT include hand washing clothes, hanging them out on a clothes line, vacuuming the house, gardening and washing the car. NEAT is really any energy that we expend outside vigorous structured, planned exercise such as a daily run or going to the gym to lift weights or use the chair climber.

Dr. Levine developed and utilized state of the art measuring devices in his studies of people's everyday activities, and he has determined that people who are able to maintain a healthy body weight expend approximately 2.5 hours more NEAT per day than people who have difficulty maintaining their weight.[7]

Dr. Levine has commented, "Thus, the obesity epidemic may reflect the emergence of a chair-enticing environment to which those with an innate tendency to sit, did so, and became obese. To reverse obesity, we need to develop individual strategies to promote standing and ambulating time by 2.5 hours/day and also re-engineer our work, school, and home environments to render active living the option of choice."

Why is NEAT more helpful in maintaining weight than structured exercise? Because we perform NEAT more often! We do NEAT 7 days a week every day of the year. Most people only perform structured exercise three or four times a week. This is diagrammed in the following figure.

In the figure, several examples of energy expenditure are given for the same-sized man. The men have the same body shape and equivalent basal metabolic rates (blue portion of bars—BMR-energy expended daily to keep basic body functions running, such as breathing, pumping blood, and neurons firing). The blue-collar worker (Everyday Moderate Exercise) expends more energy per day in NEAT (green portion of bars) than the worker (Sedentary) who sits at a desk all day. Even adding 1 hour of walking per day (300 kcal; red portion of bar) or 1 hour of swimming per day (425 kcal; yellow portion of bar) to the desk worker's total energy expenditure does not bring the total kilocalories expended for the day by the desk worker up to

---

[7] Levine JA, Vander Weg MW, Hill JO, Klesges RC (2006). Non-exercise activity thermogenesis: The crouching tiger hidden dragon of societal weight gain. *Arteriosclerosis, Thrombosis and Vascular Biology* 26: 729–736. http://atvb.ahajournals.org/content/26/4/729.long

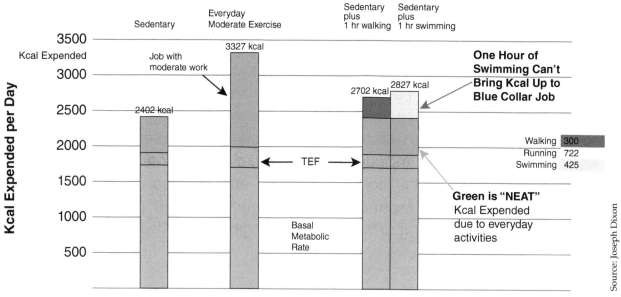

Source: Joseph Dixon

Example where 1 hour of structured exercise per day cannot make up for loss of expenditure activity during a day's work that includes moderate to heavy physical activity. The kilocalorie per hour expended in three types of activities is shown on the right. One hour of walking would add 300 kcal, 1 hour of swimming would add 425 kcal, and 1 hour of running would add 722 kcal to the energy expended by the man with the desk job. Most energy is expended by the Basal Metabolic Rate (Blue). The Orange portion is the energy expended by the thermic effect of food (TEF), which is due to digestion and distribution of food nutrients. The green region is energy expended in physical activity—most of it coming from NEAT.

the amount of energy expended by the blue-collar worker. An hour of running per day (722 kcal) might equalize the number of Calories burned to that of the blue-collar worker.

Most people who perform structured exercise regularly do so only about 4 hours per week or less. People who perform greater than average NEAT do so every day/7 days a week! On average, a person who expends a large amount of kilocalories in everyday activities will burn 500 more kcal/day than a person with a similar body type who does little NEAT per day. The reason for our lower levels of NEAT today are due to many reasons—jobs where we sit all day in front of a computer, no need to hand wash the clothes and hang them out to dry, driving to the supermarket instead of walking or having to hitch the horse to the buggy. The reasons are numerous because of all the work saving devices that have been introduced into modern day society. The introduction into the home of the two major digital systems in the late 1900s: (1) cable TV, large screen televisions, VCRs, and the remote control devices that led to longer hours of inactivity, and (2) easy to use and more powerful desktop computers, and later laptops, that also kept people stationary in chairs.

Dr. James Levine, in a series of illuminating studies, documented the role of NEAT (i.e., the lack of it) in the obesity crisis in the U.S. And it turned out that the time people spent in everyday activities contributed more energy expenditure than the time they spent in the gym in their new cross trainer shoes. See his articles through the links below!

How Do We Increase NEAT in Our Everyday Lives?

It's easy—but hard. By this I mean all we have to do is to reverse what we have done to decrease NEAT in the past 100 years. But giving up our digital devices and other work savers requires a conscious decision not to benefit from all of these modern conveniences. Here are some suggestions. The first thing to do is to throw out the television set. There is nothing that causes you to sit and not move more than watching television. If you do not wish to part with your TV, then an alternate would be to throw out the couch and replace it with a treadmill. However, most people do not use their treadmills no matter what! Another way to increase NEAT is sell the car and to walk to work and/or use public transportation. This will provide 30 to 90 min/day of exercise depending upon the circumstances of your commute. If it is impossible to commute to work from where you live—move! And the act of moving will boost your activity level right there and then! Another way to increase NEAT is to get a job where you need to walk around. Again, you need to be committed in order to get that NEAT! If you do not want to change jobs, consider installing a treadmill desk in your office. In fact, there are directions on how to build your own treadmill desk on the internet! And you can get exercise in the building process! There are numerous ways to increase NEAT in your life!

Much of the above suggestions are extreme, but the benefits of getting more NEAT are worth it. With more NEAT, slowly that weight will come off, and you will start to feel the muscles throughout your body become more firm. You will feel better and be able to keep up with your younger companions. And as you lose weight, your blood lipids and glucose will improve, too.

What is structured exercise good for? It is incredibly important in the long term!

Yes, it is amazingly important because you still need the four health benefits that I wrote about earlier in this chapter. Most important, you need to perform 4 hours of strenuous exercise per week, in addition to the increased NEAT, to keep your heart muscles and coronary artery smooth muscle cells in good shape!

Please see a few of the many publications by Dr. James Levine by clicking on the links below:

http://bjsm.bmj.com/content/41/9/558.long#global-tab-quality

http://www.hindawi.com/journals/jobe/2011/358205/

My Personal Battle with NEAT

For many people who have jobs in the information services, the opportunity to move during our job has been greatly reduced. One way that I have increased my NEAT is to walk and take the train to work. This is not an easy decision to make. If I take the car, I can make it door to door in about 15 minutes. But if I walk and take the train, the trip can take up to 1.5 hours. But the rewards are many. For example, in walking to the train station, I can think about the coming day and make plans. Some of the best ideas I have formulated have occurred while walking. Then at the train station, I walk down a series of steps and then walk up a similar series of steps.

My legs and knees always feel better after having done this. Then it is time to wait on the platform. In the morning this is often done with the sun shining on my face and hands. I can feel those photons penetrating my skin making vitamin D out of skin cholesterol. Then the train comes and there is always something exciting about getting on a train. During the short trip to New Brunswick, I get to see all the people on the train, and I guarantee you that the infinite variety of people on the train is always interesting.

Then it is time to walk about a block to wait for the bus. It is not as exciting as the train, but the bus is still highly entertaining as 90% of the passengers are students, some of whom I have had in my classes. Finally, it is about a two-block walk to my building. When I sit down at my desk, I am much more prepared to start the day after having taken public transportation compared to when I drive. I have maybe seen 30 or 40 people up close. It just feels more like a "village." Whereas when I drive I become stressed out by all the bad drivers on the road—those talking on the phone while driving; those putting on their makeup while driving, and worst of all, those texting while driving. When I drive, by the time I arrive at my building, I am already shaken and stressed out from fighting off a hundred or so other bad drivers on the road. My blood pressure must be about 20 points higher when I drive to work.

Therefore, the benefits to health of walking and taking mass transportation to work are many and include keeping the NEAT up and having extra time to enjoy the trip rather than becoming angry as your fight off the other drivers on the road. Of course the down side is the extra time it takes to get to work and every once in a while you forget your umbrella and get a little wet along the way. Also, in the era of worries about being close to other travelers, as in the COVID-19 pandemic of 2020, one might wish to avoid public transportation to prevent catching an infectious disease.

Overall Summary

If you have fallen into the habit of not exercising for many years, and if you spend a great deal of time on the couch watching TV, you will need to change your basic way of living. A classic diet alone won't help! If you have already gained weight so that you are overweight or obese, you will need to increase your NEAT by about 2 and half hours a day. It may take several years, but this will help with weight control. But most importantly, your philosophy during this time of smarter eating and increased NEAT is that you are making these changes to become healthier!

Why Classic Diets Fail!

There are thousands of books on diets (called "Classic" Diets in this book) to lose weight, and each diet is usually called a different name. In reality, there is only a small group of diets possible, and most experts do not recommend those that call for an extreme change in the macronutrient content. Instead, academic scientists and Registered Dietitians recommend a comprehensive change in lifestyle, with healthy eating being just one aspect of a healthy lifestyle. This chapter will discuss the major Classic diets, how they are supposed to work, and why they fail.

The major theme of this book is that the Obesity Explosion was the result of multilevel changes in our postindustrial, post-food–engineered, and postdigital world. So many books out there have as their premise that just making a few changes in your diet (in other words, following the Classic diet approach[1]) will propel you to lose weight, and become the person you wish to be. It is obvious from the arguments I present in this book that I feel this kind of approach will not meet with success. The changing of one factor (the diet) is bound not to be powerful enough for consistent and permanent weight loss when so many other parts of the environment you live in are stacked against you regarding weight loss and health.

So in a discussion of diets, it is first fruitful to discuss why diets alone will not work, and, in some cases, explain why the internet/Classic diet approach may even lead to greater weight gain. Dr. Charlotte Markey, Chairman of the Department of Psychology at Rutgers University-Camden, has written a book,

---

[1] A Classic diet is defined as following a prescribed set of instructions that dictates the limits to what foods or macronutrients can be eaten, and possibly, the particular way a food should be eaten and when. In most cases, Classic diets change only one aspect of your diet or life, and rely upon your basic psychological makeup to stay on the diet, which usually is extremely difficult and a highly artificial approach to health and life as it is actually lived. For the remainder of the chapter, these diets will be called "Classic diets" without the quotation marks.

Smart People Don't Diet,[2] which draws on results from social and psychological studies to present the argument that the Classic diet approach is a poor option for successful, sustained weight loss.

The points Dr. Markey made in her book why classic diets do not work are based on psychological principles that have to do with human brain circuitry, and are summed up as follows:

1. Enjoyment—Humans strive for enjoyment. Dieting makes you cranky! First you become hopeful, and then when you begin to slip, you become cranky! It is impossible to enjoy life on a classic diet.

2. Rebound Effects—Classic diets can actually lead to weight gain! If a diet does not work, the person often blames his or her self. There can be a significant rebound. People want what is forbidden—as Mark Train said, "There is a charm about the forbidden that makes it unspeakably desirable."

3. Body Hate is a Counterproductive Motivator—Some people feel ashamed when they compare themselves to what is considered perfection as seen on television or in magazines. Humans are not perfect. Dieters who fail several times will feel especially awful. They should always be given support and hope.

4. Dieting uses Brain Bandwidth—meaning it requires time and concentration, and when carried to an extreme, it can lead to an eating disorder. This is especially important in young girls who need to focus on school and positive life events. It is also important for adults too! When there are too many things on your mind—your efficiency slows down!

5. The psychological concept, Ironic Processing—Following a classic diet may lead to Ironic Processing—The attempt to suppress a thought makes you think about the thought!

6. "What the Hell Concept!" After you eat one of the forbidden foods like a frosted doughnut—you realize you broke the rules of the classic diet—then you say, "What the Hell," and then you eat the rest of the donuts in the package. Each of us has experienced a "What the Hell" moment.

7. Reward Theory—Humans like and respond to rewards! Some indulgence is good for your mind. It is more effective to think about caloric intake over a month's time, and then you can schedule times of reward and relaxation of rules! Reward theory has been shown to be a very powerful way to get humans to do something! (I also call it the Jolly Rancher Effect!) So it is

---

[2] Markey CN (2014). *Smart People Don't Diet.* Philadelphia, PA: Da Capo Press (Perseus Book Group).

important to provide rewards rather than negative consequences. Always schedule a break where you can enjoy a treat and not feel guilty.

8. Early Success Dooms Continued Success—Extreme Classic diets do not work in the long term—if you have early success, you may think the problem is solved—but then motivation and adherence goes away and you slowly crawl back to old habits—the rebound discussed above has started.

9. Cycling in and out of Classic diets leads to a "Cycle of False Hopes"—leading to psychological consequences such as loss of hope (see section below).

10. Energy Levels are Important in Your Life—Classic diets lower your "pep" level and metabolism. The body fights to maintain its energy stores and lowers your energy expenditure in response to Classic dieting. This is why a healthy lifestyle needs to be adopted and followed over the long term.

Consequences of Failing Over and Over with a Classic Diet

An article by Janet Polivy and C. Peter Herman[3] explored why people tend to fail when they diet, and what were the consequences when a person failed a number of times. It starts out with a dieter's desire to lose weight, but in the end, after going on a Classic diet, their expectations are usually unfulfilled. As reported in a wide number of journal articles, Classic diets are not effective ways to permanently lose weight, and 95% of those who lose weight will regain it. One problem with Classic diets is that, at first, they usually do succeed, but as the person loses interest or goes off the diet, he or she begins to regain the weight. People get their hopes up that they will quickly be successful, and then when progress slows, they become discouraged. So people who go on classic diets start off with high expectations for weight loss, but if and when they fail, they need to blame something, so they often blame themselves. Another scenario involves people who feel, from the beginning, that they will never be successful, and they only go into a diet half-heartedly, and of course, little progress is made.

So why do people wish to diet in the first place?? Most people wish to improve their lives. People envision rewards from losing weight, such as getting a better job or entering into a new romance. They wish to look like a thinner version of himself or herself. They believe losing weight will make them happy.

---

[3] Polivy J, Herman CP (2002). If at first you don't succeed. False hopes of self-change. *Am Psychol* 57(9): 677–689. https://www.ncbi.nlm.nih.gov/pubmed/12237978

So why do diets fail? There are many reasons. Classic diets require one to be in control, but most of us can never stay in control of ourselves for every minute. Diets often involve negative thinking—I can't have this; I can't have that. This negative thinking is very destructive—especially when it involves multiple attempts at dieting. Cycling through "the false hope syndrome" leads to medical problems and "negative psychological consequences."[4] There are multiple consequences to dieting: obsession, anxiety, irritation, depression.

In fact, the whole beriberi, "I can't, I can't," concept of classic dieting is wrong psychologically. A major psychological fact is that humans respond highly to positive reinforcement. So to be halfway successful, diets should inhabit a positive, brighter plane: I am looking forward to this and that, and then once a week, I can have a reward. Classic diets should be easy, fun, and doable, but they never are—they take too much energy, and time.

So what can dieters do? First, dieters need to become comfortable and happy with themselves. This is the key to living a fulfilled life. There are many books on this. Two resources are: a website by Dr. Robert Waldinger, who was director of the Harvard Study of Adult Development,[5] and a book from this study.[6] Second, reasonable goals need to be set. In the short term, major losses in weight are not possible—biology will not allow it. If someone gained weight over 10 to 15 years, it is not going to come off in 3 months, or even 6 months. But long term, one can morph into a healthier person in several different ways. In the long term, with solid knowledge, self-change is possible. But it requires time and a new way of looking at eating and health.

Classic Diets Are Almost Always Based Upon a Few Variants That Have Been Shown to be Unhelpful, and Often, Unhealthy

Let's dive deeper into Classic diets. There are thousands of books that have a certain media diet as their entire subject. I have dedicated just this one chapter to diets, for the basic reason that all diet books, and all popular diets, are derivatives of a very few number of diet possibilities (or variants). The diet possibilities are:

1. Extreme macronutrient distribution diets
2. Inclusion or exclusion diets

---

[4] Foreyt JP, Brunner RL, Goodrick GK, Cutter G, Brownell KD, St Jeor ST (1995). Psychological correlates of weight fluctuation. *Int J Eat Disorders* 17(3): 263–275. https://www.ncbi.nlm.nih.gov/pubmed/7773263

[5] http://adultdevelopment.wix.com/harvardstudy

[6] George E. Vaillant MD (2003) *Aging Well: Surprising Guideposts to a Happier Life from the Landmark Harvard Study of Adult Development*. Little, Brown Spark.

3. Very–low-calorie diets (often a liquid diet)
4. Diets with external structural support (usually diets that one pays for)
5. Diets that use eccentric, or bizarre preparation techniques (e.g., The Paleo diet)

Because all media diets are based on a few very simple variations of the basic average American diet, the diets that have been recently popularized have actually been around for 70 years or more, and every so often, they erupt with renewed popularity. A book by Theodore Berland, *Rating the Diets,* was published in 1975 and is still the best review of diets ever written.[7] It is 100% pertinent today, and in my mind, it is the most informative book concerning specific diets. This guide reviews, in detail, many popular diets, including Dr. Atkin's, Dr. Stillman's, Mayo, Prudent, Zen, Kennedy Hormone Diet Program, Cellulite Diet, Boston Police Diet, and many other diets. *Rating the Diets,* by the former Chicago Tribune health columnist, Theodore Berland, is extremely well written and comprehensive. It is also extensively referenced with early scientific articles describing studies of many of these diets. Many of these articles, like the book, have been forgotten, but they are still relevant and scientifically pertinent.

The Carousel of Popular Diets

In the next table, I have compared the different main diets that rely on variations in macronutrient content that are popular today. In the left most column is the typical American diet as recently determined by the USDA. The typical American diet shown is an amalgam of many diets consumed in the United States. This diet is also called the "Western Diet". In the second column is the low-carbohydrate diet (Low Carb Diet) that is also called the Atkins Diet. In the middle column is the Zone high protein diet that many students in my class who are weight training adhere to. The fourth column is the very–low-fat diet (also known as the Dean Ornish diet), which is essentially a high complex carbohydrate diet as it contains high amounts of unprocessed carbohydrates (i.e., it contains principal starches as eaten throughout early agriculture). And the fifth diet is the Mediterranean diet, which was first proposed and written about by Dr. Ancel Keys.[8]

---

[7] Berland, Theodore, and the Editors of Consumer Guide. (1975). *Rating the Diets.* Consumer Guide (Stokie, Illinois), Volume 77, April.

[8] Keys A, Keys M (1975). *How to Eat Well and Stay Well the Mediterranean Way.* Garden City, New York: Doubleday & Company.

	Ave American Diet	Low-Carb Diet	High-Protein Diet	Low Fat/High Carb	Mediterranean Diet
	Varies but contains red meat, hamburgers, fried foods, cheese, butter, processed foods, vegetable oils, soda, sugar, salt, beer, baked high-carb/fat snacks	Actually, the very low carbohydrate diet; Atkins diet–less than 20 g of carbohydrate daily, with a gradual increase to 50 g daily High-fat diet–Eat all you want of meat, cheese, veggies	Zone diet–40-30-30 balance of calories from carbohydrate, fat, and protein. Limited number of high-protein foods available	Dean Ornish–Vegetarian diet containing 10% of calories from fat; Whole grains, vegetables, no meat; Low-Fat/ High-Carb (Complex) Diet!	Fish and other seafood, whole grains, nuts, many types of leaf veggies, olive oil, occasional meat, red wine, fruits and vegetables; usually low in milk and butter
Carbs Fat Protein	50% 35% 15%	5% 55–65% 20–30%	40% 30% 30%	70% 10% 20%	50% 35% 15%
Negatives	High sugar, fat, salt, low in fiber Processed foods tend to have hidden kcal	Too little carb to keep glycogen up; exercise may suffer **Very–high-fat diet;** *Very* difficult to stay on for long periods	Hard to consistently eat high protein Can't do without supplements; Expensive	Very hard to stay on; Low satiety Some people sensitive to high carbs-hyperTG	Need access to fresh produce and seafood; ingredients may be expensive, Need time to prepare
Positives	None. Has led to the Obesity Explosion	Sometimes rapid initial weight loss–attributed to loss of water early on Some people like this diet	Enough Carbs to maintain glycogen; More balanced than Low-Carb diet	Some people with high LDL respond well to Ornish Diet High fiber, plant proteins predominate	High fiber; clinical Trial confirmed decrease in CHD
kcal Intake Goal to Lose Wt	No Goal	Goal: Kcal per day do not have to decrease; Allowed foods unrestricted But often kcal intake is way lower	Goal: 300 kcal/day lower than maintenance kcal intake	Goal: 300 kcal/day lower than maintenance kcal intake	Goal: Concept of healthy diet and lifestyle

Source: Joseph Dixon

In my opinion, all diets are viable if they are healthy—for both the short term and the long term. Also, all healthy diets could conceivably work, if they are coupled with major changes in lifestyle. People are different and they tend to gravitate to diets that fit their lifestyle and basic tendencies. But I will only address the popular diets that are based on altering the macronutrient levels, as these are the ones that are most often written about in trade books and in magazine articles.

The Average American Diet

The average American diet is the diet many Americans, but not all, eat. Since there are 330 million Americans, it is impossible to come up with a diet that is consumed by all or most Americans. However, we know from national studies that the breakdown of where dietary Calories come from, on average, is pretty close to the following: 50% of Calories are supplied by carbohydrates of all types, 35% of Calories are supplied by fats of all types, and 15% of Calories are supplied by proteins of all types. We know from visiting major supermarkets all around the country that very popular items that are sold in large quantities are breads made with refined flour, snack foods made with refined grains, pastas and rice, vegetable oils from many different plant sources, and foods with concentrated sources of protein, such as meat, fish, and processed meat products. In most large supermarkets, there are now several store length aisles with freezer cases containing processed foods of many kinds, including frozen pizzas, prepared foods, vegetables, and sweet concoctions of every kind containing dairy fats, sugar, synthetic and natural flavors. Almost all frozen foods (except rapidly frozen vegetables) contain added sodium in order to camouflage the well-recognized, and negatively connoting, frozen food taste.

The Low-Carbohydrate Diet

The low-carbohydrate (Low Carb) diet has been around for many years (it was discussed at length in Theodore Berland's 1975 book), but it has recently become popular again. It is predicated on the concept that high intakes of carbohydrates are obesogenic because they lead to an increased insulin level, which supports energy storage over utilization, whereas the opposite situation, intakes of extremely low-carbohydrate diets, prevents this. This is a complex metabolic issue and I will not discuss this in depth. However, in two recent studies of patients fed low-carbohydrate diets in a metabolic ward, there was less loss of body fat on low-carbohydrate diets compared to isocaloric (containing similar Calories) high-carbohydrate diets. In the first study, low carbohydrate led to less daily energy expenditure.[9] In the second study, a very–low-carbohydrate diet led to a very small, insignificant increase in daily energy expenditure (57 kcal/day).[10]

A very important distinction here is that I am talking about the very–low-carbohydrate diet, where carbohydrate intake is at first set at 20 g/day, which computes to just 80 kcal out of entire intake of 2,000 kcal, or less than 5% of the total kilocalorie intake. And then carbohydrate intake is increased gradually up to 50 g of carbohydrate, and at this level, carbohydrate intake makes up only about 10% of total kilocalorie intake. This compares to the 50% of total kilocalorie intake that carbohydrates provide in the typical American diet. Because carbohydrates are so low in this diet, the very–low-carbohydrate diet is actually a high-fat diet! You have to get your calories from somewhere! But most nutritionists feel that if a very–low-carbohydrate diet actually works (due to the fact that the person adheres to it very closely), it works because most kilocalories in our diet are supplied by carbohydrates, and when you eliminate carbohydrates, you eliminate total kilocalories from the diet. Therefore, lower-energy intake can occur on very–low-carbohydrate diet! I have known several colleagues who like and prefer the very–low-carbohydrate diet and have used it to lose weight. They will follow the low-carbohydrate diet for a couple of weeks and then cycle back onto their regular diet. Then a few months later, or when they feel they are gaining weight, they go back on the very–low-carbohydrate diet. Therefore, if the low-carbohydrate diet appeals to someone, I applaud their use of this diet. But it is important to know what is going on metabolically.

Dr. John Yudan, M.D., who was a Professor of Nutrition at the University of London, and who was a proponent of removing as much sugar from the diet as possible, commented in 1960, "We now also understand why this diet can lead to loss of weight in the obese. It is low in Calories, and it is this which causes loss of weight, and not some peculiarity in carbohydrates metabolism."[11]

The negatives and positives of the very–low-carbohydrate diet are listed in the table above.

---

[9] Hall KD, Bemis T, Brychta R, Chen KY, Courville A, Crayner EJ, Goodwin S, Guo J, Howard L, Knuth ND, Miller BV 3rd, Prado CM, Siervo M, Skarulis MC, Walter M, Walter PJ, Yannai L (2015). Calorie for calorie, dietary fat restriction results in more body fat loss than carbohydrate restriction in people with obesity. *Cell Metabol* 22(3): 427–436. https://www.ncbi.nlm.nih.gov/pubmed/26278052

[10] Hall KD, Chen KY, Guo J, Lam YY, Leibel RL, Mayer LE, Reitman ML, Rosenbaum M, Smith SR, Walsh BT, Ravussin E (2016). Energy expenditure and body composition changes after an isocaloric ketogenic diet in overweight and obese men. *Am J Clinical Nutrition* 104(2): 324–333. https://www.ncbi.nlm.nih.gov/pubmed/27385608

[11] Yudan J, Carey M (1960). The treatment of obesity by the High-fat diet—the inevitability of calories. *Lancet* (Oct 29, 1960), pp. 939–941. http://www.ncbi.nlm.nih.gov/pubmed/?term=The+treatment+of+obesity+by+the+High-fat+diet+%E2%80%93+the+inevitability+of+calories

Zone, High-Protein Diet

The high-protein diet provides at least 30% of kilocalories from protein and if possible—more. Consuming 30% of kilocalories from protein sounds reasonable, but in reality, it is difficult to obtain this much protein in the diet due to the naturally low content of protein in most foods (ranging between 11% and 16% of kilocalories in foods). Another difficulty is that there is a limited number of protein-rich foods, which leads to boredom when eating the high-protein diet. However, with time more and more high-protein foods are appearing in supermarkets. Also, a protein supplement often needs to be consumed to reach the 30% of kilocalories from protein level. The biggest plus of the classic high-protein diet is that there are ample carbohydrate kilocalories in this diet (40% of Calories from carbohydrates) that can be used for energy and to restock glycogen stores.

Low-Fat/High-Carbohydrate Diet

The very–low-fat/high-carbohydrate diet is supported by several well-respected medical authorities (including Dr. Dean Ornish) for the treatment and prevention of cardiovascular diseases such as CHD. Because this diet only contains about 10% of kilocalories from fat, the majority of kilocalories must be provided by carbohydrates. Therefore, the low-fat diet is, in fact, a high-carbohydrate diet. But the carbohydrates are derived from wholegrain products, and therefore, this is similar to what humans ate for 10,000 years during early agriculture. Also, there is high intake of fruits and vegetables, so this diet also contains high fiber. Because of the composition of the diet, it is nutrient dense. The main problem with the low-fat/high-carbohydrate diet is that it provides low satiety due to the low-fat content in the diet. Therefore, although there is no doubt that it is a heart healthy diet, it is difficult for many people to stay on the very–low-fat/high-carbohydrate diet. However, there are certain people who enjoy this diet and remain on it for their entire adult lives. It helps if one stops shopping in a conventional supermarket. Because this diet contains little fat, one must learn to cook in such a way that low-fat foods remain tasty and exciting.

The Mediterranean Diet (will be Covered in a Separate Chapter)

The Mediterranean diet is in the far right column in the table, and this diet was promoted in Ancel and Margaret Keys' cookbook, *How to Eat Well and Stay Well the*

Mediterranean Way.[12,13] I will discuss the Mediterranean Diet in detail in the next chapter of this book. But if you look through the extensive table, you will see that the Mediterranean diet maintains the approximate macro nutrient percentages of the typical American diet, but the ingredients and methods of food preparation are totally different. An important aspect of the Mediterranean diet is that it is a high-fiber diet. Also, a recently published clinical trial confirmed that the Mediterranean diet was protective against diseases of the heart. But most importantly, the Mediterranean diet includes changes in lifestyle that are important and make it even more effective.

A study that investigated which of the Previous Diets was best for losing weight

Let's discuss a study that tested several important Classic diets.[14]

Dansinger et al. tested four diets to investigate which diet was best for losing weight, and which diet was adhered to best over the course of a year. Below are three of the diets studied; the fourth was the Weight Watches diet, which is a commercial diet that has evolved since the study was conducted.

Atkins diet—Start with less than 20 g of carbohydrate daily, with a gradual increase towards 50 g daily. (Also called **Very–Low-Carb Diet!**)

Zone diet—40-30-30 balance of percentage calories from carbohydrate, fat, and protein. (Also called the **High-Protein Diet!**)

Dean Ornish diet—Vegetarian diet developed by **Dr. Dean Ornish** containing 10% of calories from fat. (Also called the **Low-Fat/High-Carb [Complex] Diet!**)

Study Design. The study was a 1-year randomized trial of the dietary components of the Atkins, Zone, and Ornish diets. Participants (160 individuals, about 50:50 men:women) were enrolled in the study conducted in Boston, MA. Each group contained about 40 individuals. Enrollees were adults of any age who were overweight or obese with a body mass index between 27 and 42. Each participant

---

[12] Keys A, Keys M (1975). *How to Eat Well and Stay Well the Mediterranean Way.* Garden City, New York: Doubleday & Company.

[13] Dixon JL (2015). *Genius and Partnership: Ancel and Margaret Keys and the Discovery of the Mediterranean Diet.* New Brunswick, NJ: Joseph L Dixon Publishing.

[14] Dansinger ML, Gleason JA, Griffith JL, Selker HP, Schaefer EJ (2005). Comparison of the Atkins, Ornish, Weight Watchers, and Zone diets for weight loss and heart disease risk reduction: a randomized trial. *JAMA* 293(1): 43–53. http://jama.jamanetwork.com/article.aspx?articleid=200094

had to have at least one metabolic cardiac risk factor in order to provide motivation for finishing the study.

The participants were taught the diets through 1-hour meetings on four occasions during the first 2 months of the study. A dietitian and physician described the diets and gave general advice on how to adhere to each diet. Written materials and an official diet cookbook were given to each participant. During the course of the study, food intake was monitored using 3-day food records at baseline, 1, 2, 6, and 12 months.

Results of the Study

After a year in the study, the mean weight loss was similar across all the diets. At 1 year, weight loss averaged about 2 to 3 kg/person, or only a mean weight loss of about 2% to 3%. Also, the 1-year discontinuation rates were: Atkins, 48% stopped; Ornish, 50% stopped; and Zone diet, 35% stopped. So the Atkins and Ornish diets appeared harder to stay on, and more people adhered to the Zone high-protein diet. The above weight loss figures were means for the groups. However, individuals did have successes. Three individuals on the Ornish diet and one person on the Zone diet lost more than 20 kg of body weight, whereas no one on the Atkin's diet lost this much weight after 1 year in the study.

The conclusions from the study by Dansinger et al. were[15]:

"Our findings challenge the concept that 1 type of diet is best for everybody and that alternative diets can be disregarded."

"…our findings do not support the notion that very–low-carbohydrate diets are better than standard diets, despite recent evidence to the contrary."

"…poor sustainability and adherence rates resulted in modest weight loss and cardiac risk factor reductions for each diet group…"

Overall Conclusions

Unless one adheres to a diet, the diet will not succeed, no matter which diet is chosen. The psychological makeup of the individual is as important to the success of a diet as the particular diet being tried.

Therefore, one must conclude that rather than following a prescribed diet, one might be more successful if he or she switched to a healthy lifestyle! This was the exact conclusion that Ancel and Margaret Keys came to when they wrote their

---

[15] Dansinger ML, et al. (2005), Ibid, See conclusions.

book, *"How to Eat Well and Stay Well the Mediterranean Way,"* published by Doubleday in 1975.

Next, the Best Diet to Follow for General Health, for Prevention of Coronary Heart Disease, and for Combating Obesity—The Mediterranean Diet, First Championed by Dr. Ancel Keys and his Chemist Spouse, Margaret!

The Healthy Mediterranean Diet

In the 1950s, Ancel and Margaret Keys set out on a worldwide trek to discover why Americans, and people of a few other developed countries, exhibited high rates of heart attacks compared to everyone else. In their travels they came across the diet of the Italian people, who at that time exhibited almost no CHD in their population. The Keyses published a book in 1959 about the healthy diet they observed in Italy and the other Mediterranean countries they visited. In 1975, the Keyses published an updated version of their book–called, *How to Eat Well and Stay Well the Mediterranean Way.*

The Mediterranean diet is more than a diet. Rather, it encompasses a way of life that is lived over a long period of time and includes daily routines such as walking, shopping for healthy foods, cooking, eating Mediterranean foods, enjoying life, and having a calm and moderate outlook and philosophy. For all intents and purposes, the Mediterranean diet came to prominence when Ancel Keys started the Seven Countries Study in the mid to late 1950s for the purpose of finding out why American men were succumbing to CHD at much greater rates than men in some countries in southern Europe. When Dr. Keys and wife Margaret, a laboratory chemist, first visited Naples, Italy, in the mid-1950s, they were astounded how few cases of CHD could be found in the local hospitals. They wondered the reason for this, and because at the time, not that long after World War II, the diet of the inhabitants of this area of Italy was largely made of vegetable based foods, especially many different types of green leafy lettuces and other vegetables of an extremely wide variety. But CHD and high blood pressure are complex diseases, so Dr. Keys assembled a team of international doctors and nutritionists to study the influence of diet on the cardiovascular system, and this study was to become known as the Seven Countries study. For the full story of how the Seven Countries Study was designed and implemented, please read my book: *Genius and Partnership: Ancel and Margaret Keys and the Discovery of the Mediterranean Diet.*[1]

Summary of the Seven Countries Study

The Seven Countries study was a massive study (and, for that time, totally unprecedented) that followed 12,763 men, aged 40 to 59, from seven countries with wide contrasts in traditional diet: Finland, Greece, Italy, Japan, the Netherlands, the United States, and Yugoslavia. The overall findings (from many published books and articles) of these studies, including the 10-year follow-up of the participants who were recruited, were published in a book, *Seven Countries*, by Ancel Keys et al. (1980).[2] However, the Seven Countries study is still going on today as the analysis of the 50-year data of the few men surviving from the original study were published recently.[3]

The main conclusions of the Seven Countries study, presented in the 1980 book, were: "Our ten year finding, and concordance with other studies, make it clear that the big three risk factors for coronary heart disease now established are age, blood pressure, and serum cholesterol."[4]

Today these conclusions seem unremarkable. However, at the time, they were earth-shattering findings (except for the age factor) and, in fact, they had very significant effects on the American population as CHD rates dropped in the U.S. in the second half of the 1900s.

The overall results of Seven Countries were very influential as many men who would have died in their 40s and 50s of heart attacks, lived much longer, into their 70s and 80s. My father had his first attack at the age of 85. Many of us have benefited greatly by having our fathers and mothers live much longer because Ancel Keys and his colleagues pursued the mystery of the effects of diet on CVD.

In addition to the Seven Countries study, which was a multi country, epidemiological study, Dr. Keys also carried out about 25 years of human feeding trials in his laboratory at the University of Minnesota.

---

[1] Dixon JL (2015). *Genius and Partnership: Ancel and Margaret Keys and the Discovery of the Mediterranean Diet.* New Brunswick, NJ: Joseph L. Dixon Publishing.

[2] Keys A, Aravanis C, Blackburn H, Buzina R, Djordjević BS, Dontas AS, Fidanza F, Karvonen MJ, Kimura N, Menotti A, Mohacek I, Nedeljković S, Puddu V, Punsar S, Taylor HL, Van Buchem FSP (1980). *Seven Countries: A Multivariate Analysis of Death and Coronary Heart Disease.* Cambridge, MA: Harvard University Press, ISBN: 0-674-80237-3, 381 pp.

[3] Kromhout D, Menotti A, Alberti-Fidanza A, Puddu PE, Hollman P, Kafatos A, Tolonen H, Adachi H, Jacobs DR Jr (2018). Comparative ecologic relationships of saturated fat, sucrose, food groups, and a Mediterranean food pattern score to 50-year coronary heart disease mortality rates among 16 cohorts of the Seven Countries Study. *Eur J Clin Nutr* 72(8): 1103–1110. doi: 10.1038/s41430-018-0183-1. https://www.ncbi.nlm.nih.gov/pubmed/29769748

[4] Keys A, et al. (1980). Ibid, p. 341.

In 1960, Dr. Keys and his laboratory group published a very interesting feeding study in the *Journal of Nutrition* that investigated the effects of a typical "American" diet of the time versus a typical "Italian" diet.[5] The diets contained precisely controlled fat contents of either low- or moderate-fat levels. But the diets varied greatly in the amount of vegetables and meat that were included. And the blood cholesterol values were much lower when the men consumed the "Italian" diet. What is interesting is that Dr. Keys did not yet label the "Italian" diet he was testing the "Mediterranean" diet. That would come later, when he and Margaret published their third cooking and health book, *How to Eat Well and Stay Well the Mediterranean Way*.

The upshot of all this is that the many publications that resulted from the Seven Countries study, and the feeding studies, pointed to saturated fat in the diet as being an important factor in the regulation of blood cholesterol concentrations, and it was the blood cholesterol concentration that was an important factor in the rate of CHD disease that a particular population experienced.

Dr. Keys become a proponent of the Mediterranean diet, and he and his wife, Margaret, wrote a series of bestselling cook books that described how to follow this lifestyle/diet.

These books were Eat Well and Stay Well (1959),[6] The Benevolent Bean, published in 1967,[7] and *How to Eat Well and Stay Well the Mediterranean Way*.[8] All of the books were featured on New York Times Best Seller lists.

Why Is the Mediterranean Diet the Healthiest Diet?

Although many studies have indicated that the Mediterranean diet is one of the healthiest diets, we actually don't know why. There are many theories, and the one that seems to have the most traction, is that it is a combination of factors that make it healthy. For example, in 2018, a study using 25,994 healthy U.S. women enrolled in the large Women's Health Study concluded that eating a Mediterranean diet was associated with about a 25% decrease in CVD events.[9] Consuming a more complete and comprehensive Mediterranean diet (highest one-third compared to the lowest one-third) positively

---

[5] Keys A, Anderson JT, Grande F (1960). Diet-type (fats constant) and blood lipids in man. *J Nutrition* 70: 257–266. http://jn.nutrition.org/content/70/2/257.long

[6] Keys A, Keys M (1959). *Eat Well and Stay Well*. Garden City, New York: Doubleday & Company.

[7] Keys A, Keys M (1967). *The Benevolent Bean*. Garden City, New York: Doubleday & Company. Edition read: Noonday Edition, 1972, New York: Noonday Press (a division of Farrar, Straus and Giroux).

[8] Keys A, Keys M (1975). *How to Eat Well and Stay Well the Mediterranean Way*. Garden City, New York: Doubleday & Company.

[9] Ahmad S, Moorthy MV, Demler OV, Hu FB, Ridker PM, Chasman DI, Mora S (2018). Assessment of risk factors and biomarkers associated With risk of cardiovascular disease among women consuming a Mediterranean Diet. *JAMA Netw* 1(8):e185708 https://www.ncbi.nlm.nih.gov/pubmed/30646282

affected a number of Potential Risk Mediators, such as inflammation, various lipoproteins, and insulin parameters. Although it was mentioned by the authors that food frequency questionnaires were used to assess Dietary intake, the results are in agreement with many other studies of the effects of the Mediterranean diet on Health.

But it is important to point out that the "Mediterranean diet" that Ancel and Margaret Keys observed and ate when they visited and later lived in Italy (1950s to 2000) was the one they wrote about in their books. The diet found in Mediterranean countries today has evolved somewhat since the 1950s because Italy and other countries have recovered from World War II and have become wealthier.

In Chapter 2 of their book,[10] Ancel and Margaret wrote about the foods they found in the Mediterranean countries they visited and the Mediterranean lifestyle they observed in their travels. They made the comment in the beginning of the Chapter that they were specifically talking about the countries of Greece, Italy, the Mediterranean portion of France, and Spain. Each had their own special dishes and customs. The location they knew best was southern Italy, because they decided to move to a house in the village of Pioppi, on the western coast of southern Italy, for at least 6 months of the year while Dr. Keys was still working. After he retired from the University of Minnesota in 1972, they moved there year round, and ended up living there for another 30 years.

What Was the Mediterranean Diet the Keyses Observed and Experienced?

Vegetables and Fruits

The availability of vegetables and fruits depended upon the season. Early in the spring there were cauliflower, artichokes, and lettuce available. Later, there were fava beans and a dozen different wild greens in the markets. Later still came spinach, green beans, and zucchini. Late spring brought cherries, kumquats, and mushrooms.

Summer brought figs, tomatoes, eggplants, peppers, and onions. At the end of summer, wine was prepared during the grape harvest. All sorts of melons were available in the early fall. From their own property they harvested apples, pears and a whole family of citrus fruits. Late fall saw the production of persimmons, pomegranates, and finally olives. In the end, one senses that there was a cornucopia of fresh vegetables and fruits that they were exposed to from the local farms and surrounding hillsides the year round.

---

[10] Keys A, Keys M (1975). Ibid, Chapter 2.

Olives

Olives pressed early in the season were the source of virgin olive oil. A small percentage of olives were prepared and canned for whole storage to be used as table olives during the year. The largest per capita consumption of olive oil occurred on Crete, where it provided 30% of the total caloric intake. In other areas of the Mediterranean, olive oil provided from 15% to 20% of total calories. French cooking used more butter and, therefore, was not as healthy as the cuisines of Greece and Italy.

Bread

Freshly baked bread provided a considerable amount of calories for Mediterranean peoples. Often the bread was made from locally grown and locally ground grains. In Greece, it could provide up to 38% of the total calories consumed. In other countries it was less, but it was still a significant percent of the total calories consumed. On average, at the time of Dr. Keys' investigations, three times more bread was eaten in the Mediterranean areas compared to what was eaten in the U.S.

Dessert

Fruit was the main dessert served in Mediterranean households. Sweet desserts were reserved for holidays. Peoples of the Mediterranean region ate, on average, 150% more fruit than Americans.

Garlic and Onions

These were used in cooking, stews, and salads. Garlic soup is a specialty of the Spanish whereas the French are known for their onion soup. The Italians are known for their bruschetta, which is a slice of hot toast brushed with olive oil and raw garlic.

Tomatoes and Garden Greens

The Mediterranean peoples harvested tomatoes and prepared homemade tomato sauce every August. Bottled/canned tomato sauce was used throughout the year in stews and with pastas. Also eaten all year round was a vast array of leafy greens that come from the garden or from the roadside. The Mediterranean people ate a much wider variety of greens than do Americans. These greens are high in vitamins (especially vitamin K) and minerals.

Dr. Keys wrote in a later article, "Near our second home in southern Italy, all kinds of leaves are an important part of the everyday diet. There are many kinds of lettuce, spinach, Swiss chard, purslane, and plants I cannot identify with an English name such as *lettuga, barbabietole, scarola,* and *rape.* Some are perennials. The climate permits replanting annuals several times a year so leaves to eat are always at hand. No main meal in the Mediterranean countries is replete without lots of dure (greens). *Mangiafoglia* is the Italian word for "to eat leaves" and that is a key part of the good Mediterranean diet."[11]

Seafood and Meat

Mediterranean people were strong consumers of anchovies, octopus, mackerel, dried codfish from northern seas, and a vast array of ocean fish. Fish from the Mediterranean Sea were less plentiful because the Mediterranean had been over-fished at this time.

Americans at the time (1950 and early 60s) were eating four times more meat than what was consumed in Greece and Spain. In Mediterranean countries more veal was consumed than beef, except in France. Only about half the eggs Americans ate were consumed by Mediterraneans. The French ate more butter than Americans, but the other Mediterranean countries consumed only about one-third to one-half the butter Americans did at the time.

Beverages

The consumption of wine was much greater in Mediterranean countries, but it was usually consumed with main meals. For men, the amount of wine consumed possibly amounted to about 10% of total caloric intake coming from alcohol. There was very little consumption of hard liquor except on special occasions.

The Mediterranean people are known to drink strong and freshly made coffee, often using an "espresso" machine. In fact, coffee with added hot milk was a common breakfast for Mediterranean people. Spain was the one country where people also drank a considerable amount of hot cocoa. Other drinks that were popular were lemonade, cola drinks, and mineral water. However, cola drinks were not consumed at the level consumed in the U.S. at the time.

---

[11] Keys A (1995). Mediterranean diet and public health: personal reflections. *Am J Clin Nutr.* 61(6 Suppl): 1321S–1323S. http://www.ncbi.nlm.nih.gov/pubmed/?term=7754982

The Intangibles

Mediterranean people were more likely to take an evening stroll than Americans. They were also likely to eat a wider variety of foods, especially fresh seafood and vegetables. Because of the southern sun, they received more sunlight than in northern regions on a yearly basis, and it was spread more evenly across the year. In northern regions there are periods of little sun during winter, followed by intense sun exposure during summer. In the Mediterranean regions, the exposure allowed for longer and more consistent periods of moderate vitamin D availability.

At the time Dr. Ancel Keys and Margaret wrote their Mediterranean cookbook, they commented that although the expenditures of the Mediterranean countries on health care were much less than those expended in the U.S., the Mediterranean peoples' "overall health and longevity are impressive, both in the vital statistics and in our own many years of scientific observations."[12]

The main difference in health was that there was a much lower rate of CHD in Mediterranean countries compared to the U.S. Dr. Keys specifically commented that, from his vast experience in the region, the difference was not explained by climate, genes, or the way disease was diagnosed, or how statistics were kept in the different countries. And another plus was that deaths from all causes were lower in the Mediterranean countries than in the U.S.

The remainder of the book, *How to Eat Well and Stay Well the Mediterranean Way*, is chock full of health information and recipes of all types, and as stated by the Keys in the Authors' Preface, all were tested first in their kitchens, sometimes in Pioppi, Italy, and sometimes in Minnesota, before they were entered into their cookbook.

The Keyses' books were the first ones to promote the Mediterranean diet. Combined with the early chapters on diet and health, they represent an additional major triumph in the life of this extraordinary scientist and his companion spouse.

A review article on the benefits of consuming the Mediterranean diet has recently been published.[13] The summary points from this article are the following[14]:

1. The Mediterranean diet is not a specific diet, but rather a dietary pattern followed by inhabitants of areas surrounding the Mediterranean Sea in the 1960s.

---

[12] Keys A, Keys M (1975). *How to Eat Well and Stay Well the Mediterranean Way*. Garden City, New York: Doubleday & Company, page 42.

[13] Shen J, Wilmot KA, Ghasemzadeh N, Molloy DL, Burkman G, Mekonnen G, Gongora MC, Quyyumi AA, Sperling LS (2015). Mediterranean dietary patterns and cardiovascular health. *Annual Review of Nutrition* 35: 425–449. http://www.ncbi.nlm.nih.gov/pubmed/?term=PMID%3A+++++25974696

[14] Shen J, et al. (2015). Ibid, p. 441.

2. Principles of this dietary pattern include eating an abundance of whole grains, fruits, vegetables, legumes, and nuts; using olive oil as the principal source of added fat; consuming low to moderate amounts of low-fat dairy daily; consuming a low amount of red meat; consuming a moderate amount of fish and eggs; consuming a moderate amount of wine; and using herbs and spices to flavor food.

3. Adoption of a Mediterranean dietary pattern is associated with significant reductions in serum lipids, fasting blood glucose, blood pressure, insulin resistance, arterial stiffness, and oxidative stress.

4. The Mediterranean dietary pattern is a useful tool in the primary and secondary prevention of cardiovascular disease, and its adoption has significant public health implications.

Confirmation of the Efficacy of the Mediterranean Diet for Protecting Cardiovascular Health

The Lyon Heart Study[15,16] was started in 1988 and human subjects were fed either a normal French diet or a Mediterranean diet that included a canola oil-based margarine instead of butter. The purpose of the Lyon Diet Heart study was to test the replacement of dietary saturated fat with canola oil on the incidence of primary outcomes (reinfarctions and death from heart attacks) and secondary outcomes (further CHD in myocardial infarction survivors) in patients who had suffered previous heart attacks. Six hundred and five patients were enrolled. The study was scheduled to last 5 years but was cut short after 27 months because of the highly positive effects of the canola oil group. Five hundred and eighty four subjects were included in the final analysis of the study. Myocardial infarction or death from cardiovascular disease decreased by 72% in the Mediterranean Diet group (with canola oil) compared to the Control group. Low-density lipoprotein cholesterol dropped in both groups, but interestingly, there were no differences in LDL or HDL cholesterol between the groups. The Lyon Diet Heart study showed that replacing saturated fat with polyunsaturated fat (especially moderately higher in alpha-linolenic acid and marine

[15] de Lorgeril M, Renaud S, Mamelle N, Salen P, Martin JL, Monjaud I, Guidollet J, Touboul P, Delaye J (1994). Mediterranean alpha-linolenic acid-rich diet in secondary prevention of coronary heart disease. *Lancet* 343(8911): 1454–1459. https://www.ncbi.nlm.nih.gov/pubmed/7911176

[16] de Lorgeril M, Salen P, Martin JL, Monjaud I, Delaye J, Mamelle N (1999). Mediterranean diet, traditional risk factors, and the rate of cardiovascular complications after myocardial infarction: final report of the Lyon Diet Heart Study. *Circulation* 99(6): 779–785. https://www.ncbi.nlm.nih.gov/pubmed/9989963

omega-3 fatty acids) could protect against the reoccurrence of heart attacks. The Lyon Diet Heart study is the strongest randomized clinical trial demonstrating that the Mediterranean Diet protects against CHD. Of course, the results of the Seven Countries study showed that the Mediterranean Diet was highly protective against CHD in a long-term prospective ecologic, observational epidemiological study. The 50-year follow-up study[17] showed that traditional Mediterranean and Japanese diets, rich in vegetable foods, and low in sweets and animal foods, had the lowest long-term CHD mortality rates compared to other diets.

In looking across the world at all the diets different populations consume, it is difficult to find one that is healthier than the Mediterranean diet that Ancel and Margaret Keys encountered when they visited the Mediterranean countries in the 1950s. A person who follows this diet stands a very good chance of living a long and healthy life. Dr. Ancel Keys spent a good quarter of his later years living in the village of Pioppi on the western coast of southern Italy. Possibly a combination of a healthy diet and lifestyle and good genes allowed Dr. Keys to live to be 102 years old. And most importantly, many of his later years were productive and life affirming.[18]

---

[17] Kromhout D, Menotti A, Alberti-Fidanza A, Puddu PE, Hollman P, Kafatos A, Tolonen H, Adachi H, Jacobs DR Jr (2018). Comparative ecologic relationships of saturated fat, sucrose, food groups, and a Mediterranean food pattern score to 50-year coronary heart disease mortality rates among 16 cohorts of the Seven Countries Study. *Eur J Clin Nutr* 72(8): 1103–1110. doi: 10.1038/s41430-018-0183-1. https://www.ncbi.nlm.nih.gov/pubmed/29769748

[18] Dixon JL (2015). *Genius and Partnership: Ancel and Margaret Keys and the Discovery of the Mediterranean Diet.* New Brunswick, NJ: Joseph L. Dixon Publishing.

How to Enhance the Mediterranean Diet–The Moderate Carbohydrate Intervention

> The chapter on Classic diets casts a dire shadow on the utility of these diets and their effectiveness. The Mediterranean Diet presented in the previous chapter is a tried-and-true way to achieve health and maintain weight. This chapter suggests additional strategies that may help in preventing the Obesity Explosion from becoming close and personal.

Dr. Hans Fisher's Dedication to Health

In this book I have mapped how society changed in the 1900s such that our environment became obesogenic, and therefore, the rate of obesity started to increase in the United States. In order to fight obesity, it is quite possible that each of us will need to change our everyday routine in order to remain healthy. Dr. Hans Fisher was the longest serving Professor at Rutgers University, and was also the founding chairman of the Department of Nutritional Sciences, my department at Rutgers. Dr. Fisher told me a story of how about 46 years ago, he decided that he needed to change his habits if he was going to stay healthy. He dedicated his lunch hour to working out or swimming at college pool. And therefore, no matter how important, he would not attend a meeting or talk given at noon on a workday. He also changed his diet so that he rarely ate meat. He ate mostly salads and foods that could be categorized as principal starches. One other thing—Dr. Fisher's blood cholesterol was very high and nothing he did would bring it down. When statin drugs for lowering blood cholesterol were discovered and went on the market in 1987, Dr. Fisher had his doctor immediately put him on the new medication, and they worked very well. Dr. Fisher has been on them ever since! Dr. Fisher's dedication to physical activity became well known throughout the University. Dr. Fisher retired from Rutgers University at the age of 83 years old. He had been a professor at Rutgers University for 56 years. At his current age of 90, I can assure you that Dr. Fisher is as sharp as anyone else I know, and as fit, too!

And if someone becomes overweight or obese, what actions can he or she take to regain a healthy weight? **Following Dr. Fisher's lifestyle is not a bad idea!** In the chapter on Classic diets, I presented a study performed by Michael L. Dansinger et al.,[1] who observed that after 1 year in a clinical trial, three of the most popular diets gave similar poor results concerning adherence and weight loss, mainly because people did not stay on the diets.

From this and other similar studies, the notion that has percolated up from many directions is that, "Diets do not work." But of course, this last sentence needs the following correction, "Diets do not work if you do not adhere to the diet."

But some unmistakable conclusions from the Dansinger study, and from Dr.[2] Charlotte Markey's book, are that diets are not natural, are extremely difficult to become excited about, and at the first rough period that a person encounters, the diet will be jettisoned and the person will fall back into bad habits that were followed before.

What Do I Teach in My Nutrition and Health Class about Combating Adult Obesity?

First, I teach that obesity was observed as a natural occurrence even in nonobesogenic environments, and that through evolution, a small percentage of humans, maybe 4% to 6%, were heavier than normal, and on the other end of the spectrum, about 10% of humans were extremely underweight. These individuals represent the outliers on both sides of the normal distribution of metabolic heterogeneity found in humans. This is a major strategy that has been observed over and over again in biology, and which no doubt, plays a role in survival and natural selection in humans. Some people will have a difficult time maintaining their weight even in a nonobesogenic environment and under optimal circumstances. It is just biology!

---

[1] Dansinger ML, Gleason JA, Griffith JL, Selker HP, Schaefer EJ (2005). Comparison of the Atkins, Ornish, Weight Watchers, and Zone diets for weight loss and heart disease risk reduction: a randomized trial. *JAMA* 293(1): 43–53. http://jama.jamanetwork.com/article.aspx?articleid=200094

[2] Markey CN. (2014). *Smart People Don't Diet*. Philadelphia, PA: Da Capo Press (Perseus Book Group).

The obese people are the ones who will survive the longest in a famine because of their extra energy stores. On the other hand, the people who are naturally extremely thin are able to move the fastest, and they would have the most chance of escaping a surprise attack carried out by the neighboring village.

The second point I teach is about the enormously complicated food intake regulation system that governs when and what humans eat. I present these ideas in lectures entitled, "Why Is It So Hard to Suppress Appetite?" and "How Foods Signal the Brain" (Not presented in this book). Knowing how the basic food intake regulatory system works provides students with insights into why people eat certain foods and why it is sometimes difficult to follow very subtle satiety signals. Unfortunately, the area is so complex, and there are still so many relatively unknown aspects to this field of study, that it would be impossible to address this comprehensive topic in this book.

The third point I teach in my nutrition and health class is that if you are not currently overweight and obese, you should do whatever you can to prevent weight gain from happening. The reason for this is that once a person becomes heavier than normal, the body resets its energy monitoring system, and it becomes more difficult to shed the excess weight put on.

Therefore, I am going to direct the following discussion more to how not to become obese. (Certainly, these apply widely, too)

1. Learn About Nutrition and Learn How to Cook

   The most important part of how not to become heavy is to learn about nutrition and learn how to cook nutritious and healthy foods. If you know how to cook, you never have to rely on preprepared processed foods. Of course, the students in my class are already learning about nutrition, I hope, and therefore they are already following half of this advice. The other half of this advice is an activity that one can pursue at home by following the directions of highly revered cookbooks. One I like a great deal is *The Moosewood Cookbook*, by Mollie Katzen.[3]

2. Eat Lots of Fiber

   A specific way not to become obese is to eat oatmeal (complex carbohydrate and fiber), a fruit (potassium), and a good protein (amino acids) source such as an egg for breakfast. I have recommended this to thousands of students over the years, and many have contacted me and said that they surprisingly took my advice and they believed it helped them tremendously with their health. I do not have hard data on this, but I will gladly fight anyone who thinks I am not being

---

[3] Katzen M (1992). *The Moosewood Cookbook,* Ten Speed Press, paperback, ISBN 0898154901T

absolutely truthful on this. In fact, the data on the protective properties of a high-fiber intake against coronary heart disease are incredibly strong![4]

3. Join a Food Coop

   In order to buy the ingredients that you need for the recipes in The Moosewood Cookbook, it is a great idea to join a food co-op that specializes in nonprocessed foods. In this way you will skip all the extremely unhealthy foods that you can see in the usual American supermarket. And the saying holds true—out of sight, out of mind! If you have had no prior experience preparing wholesome food, it may take a while to learn how to cook. I can vouch that you will be able to prepare every recipe in The Moosewood Cookbook with a little time and experience!

What Else can be done to Prevent Weight Gain???

One can strive to change their macronutrients—for example, decrease carbohydrates moderately by 5 to 10%, while making up the kcal by eating a little more protein and healthy fat. Is this contradictory to what I previously discussed concerning the low-carbohydrate diet? I do not think so. Below are the percentages of macronutrients in the various diets as discussed today:

Approximate Percentage of Calories coming from each macronutrient in these diets:

	Carbohydrate	Fat	Protein
Current America Diet	50%	35%	15%
Low Carbohydrate Diet	5–10%	65%	25%
Moderate Low Carbohydrate Diet	40–45%	35–40%	20%

The Moderate–Low-Carbohydrate Diet is different because it provides enough dietary carbohydrate to refill glycogen stores, but not enough to cause a spike in blood insulin after eating a meal. And the best thing about this "modification" is that it only requires you to nudge toward more healthy versions of the foods you already eat.

How to lower Carbohydrates by 5 to 10%

The way to do this without changing the basic diet you are used to is:

Eat more complex carbohydrates

---

[4] Katagiri R, Goto A, Sawada N, Yamaji T, Iwasaki M, Noda M, Iso H, Tsugane S (2020). Dietary fiber intake and total and cause-specific mortality: the Japan Public Health Center-based prospective study. *The American Journal of Clinical Nutrition* 111 (5): 1027–1035. https://academic.oup.com/ajcn/article/111/5/1027/5716885

Eat more fiber

Eat a predetermined amount of your favorite carbohydrate—use a ceremonial bowl

Cut back on sugars and other sweeteners

Avoid processed carbohydrates (essentially anything frozen)—also chips, baked goods, bread (frozen vegetable and fruits are the exceptions)

And eat carbohydrate substitutes—such as cauliflower rice for potatoes; spaghetti squash for pasta

Since 50% of the average American diet is provided by carbohydrates, then going to a moderately low-carbohydrate diet will decrease your Calorie intake. This is different than consuming a very–low-carbohydrate diet, where over the long-term people become tired of eating a very–low-carbohydrate diet. Due to our last 10,000 years of history as a society based on an agriculture model that relied mostly on principal starches, we have an innate drive for carbohydrates. Cutting down on our usual carbohydrate intake by 5% to 10% will be less likely to encounter a resistance effect.

In adolescents, going to a moderately lower-carbohydrate diet was effective in lowering liver fat. When adolescents (9 to 17 years old)[5] were given a moderately carbohydrate-restricted diet (with less than 25% of Calories from carbohydrate) for 8 weeks, liver fat decreased and insulin sensitivity improved compared to when they consumed a higher-carbohydrate diet (about 55% of Calories from carbohydrate). The moderately low-carbohydrate diet included reasonable amounts of leafy greens, nonstarchy vegetables, nuts, unsweetened yogurt, low-glycemic fruits, legumes, and small amounts of whole grains. This study highlights the utility of decreasing the carbohydrate Calories moderately instead of severely (i.e., to 5% of Calories in the diet).

Although the study by Goss et al. used an even lower-carbohydrate intake (<25% of Calories from carbohydrate), it was designed to treat a group diagnosed with nonalcoholic fatty liver disease (NAFLD). For most people lowering Calories from carbohydrate to 40% to 45% of Calories should be effective over a long period of time.

A very effective idea on how to cut down on carbohydrates in a moderate way is to obtain a ceremonial carbohydrate bowl. At every meal use this bowl to eat your carbohydrates. Fill it up and enjoy the complex carbohydrate of your choice. But except for special occasions, do not eat more complex carbohydrates than this bowl

---

[5] Goss Am, Dowla S, Pendergrass, M, Ashraf A, Bolding M, Morrison S, Amerson A, Soleymani T, Gower B (2020). Effects of a carbohydrate-restricted diet on hepatic lipid content in adolescents with non-alcoholic fatty liver disease: A pilot, randomized trial. *Pediatric Obesity* 15:e12630. https://doi.org/10.1111/ijpo.12630

can hold. A ceremonial bowl can prevent a large serving of carbohydrates scooped on a large dinner plate. See the photo of the ceremonial bowl I use in my house, placed next to some herbs from our garden.

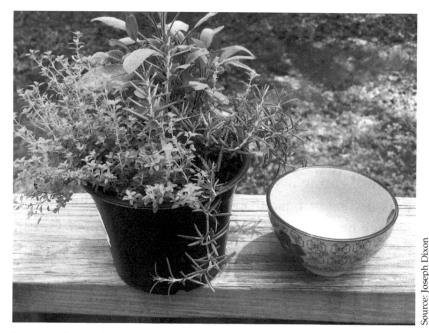

Source: Joseph Dixon

Lower Carbohydrate by 5% to 10% by Using a Ceremonial Bowl

Dietary Protein

Boost protein by 5% on a caloric basis, which for most of us, is going from about 16% of total Calorie intake from protein up to about 21% of total Calories from protein. This is not a classic diet! This is not the Zone diet that requires 30% of Calories from protein! This is just gently nudging the macronutrient breakdown a little in the direction toward protein. Why do I recommend this? I have found that I feel better after a slightly higher-protein meal. It is that simple. If I eat a very high-carbohydrate meal, either at lunch or at dinner, I want to go to sleep within about 30 minutes. Also, I find that I can exercise better after a slightly higher-protein meal eaten about 1 hour before the exercise than a meal that contains high carbohydrates. There are other benefits to a moderately high-protein diet, including increasing calcium absorption that will help maintain the density of the bones.

In the next table I show how to boost protein by 5%. The table shows the macronutrient breakdown of the American diet and then shows how to adjust the protein content of the diet. On a 2,000-kcal diet, increasing the Calories from protein by 5% is as simple as adding 25 g of protein to your diet. If you consume 3,000 kcal/day, this means you need to increase protein intake by 38 g. Today with protein bars and some high-protein foods, both of these are fairly easy to accomplish.

Macronutrient Recommendations – Based on 2000 kcal Diet

Carbohydrates	Protein	Fat
Currently % of kcal (Ave Amer) 50% kcal (2000 Total) 1000 kcal Grams 250 grams	15% 300 kcal 75 grams	35% 700 kcal 78 grams
Go to Moderate Carbohydrate Diet Decrease Carbohydrates to 40–45% % of kcal ↓ 40–45% kcal (2000 Total) ↓ to 800– 900k cal Grams 200–225 grams	Increase Protein to 20% ↑ 20% ↑ 400 kcal 100 grams	No Change – Keep Fat at 35% 35% 700 kcal 78 grams
Lower Carbohydrate kcal Intake by 5–10%: Eat as few simple sugars as possible (Do not eat processed foods) (especially chips, soda, and baked goods) Eat complex carbohydrates (principal starches) Eat as much fiber as possible from vegetables and whole grains (Frozen vegetables are fine) Use ceremonial bowl for principal starches	**Boost Protein kcal by 5%** (which is 25 grams) 3-oz Atlantic cod (19 grams of protein 3-oz steak – 24 grams of protein Smoothie with 25 grams of whey protein 6-oz canned wild Alaska salmon-36 grams of protein; 2 grams Omega 3 fatty acids (480 mg sodium (little high) **See List of High Protein foods**	**Eat mixed sources of fat** eat fish 2 times a week use healthy oils (especially olive and canola oil) eat nuts, lean meats keep dairy fat low eat canned Alaska salmon- **Get High Protein and Healthy fat in one food!!**

Source: Joseph Dixon

Also on this table is an idea how you can boost both your protein intake and snag some great omega-3 fatty acids at the same time. A 6-oz can of wild Alaska red salmon contains 36 g of protein and 2 g of omega-3 fatty acids. This food does have a fair amount of sodium (480 mg), so you may only want to eat this twice a week at most if you have blood pressure problems.

Please see the following list of foods that provide reasonable amounts of protein. And remember, this is not the Zone diet, where it is recommended by the proponents of this diet to eat 30% of total Calories from protein. The slight boost in protein that I am recommending is much easiest to attain and will provide many health benefits, including decreasing the levels of carbohydrates in the diet by a reciprocal 5% of total Calories.

In order to consume that extra 25 g of protein per day, try eating from this list of healthy and protein-rich sources (25 g of protein can be obtained by eating one or combinations of these):

3-oz steak, flank, lean, broiled—24 g of protein
3-oz chicken breast, broiled—26 g of protein
3-oz fish (flounder–broiled)—13 g of protein
3-oz Atlantic cod (broiled)—19 g of protein
4-oz tuna fish (canned in water)—26 g of protein
3-oz king salmon (kippered; canned)—24 g of protein
2 eggs—12 g of the highest-quality protein known
3.5 oz of almonds—24.9 g of protein (50 g of fat, too)
2½ protein bars (10 g protein each) (now widely available)—25 g of protein
Serving of Quinoa (1/4 cup dry) (6 g of high quality)
mixed with ½-cup cooked black beans
(7.6-g protein); Total of 13.6 g of protein
½-cup diced low-fat cheddar cheese—16 g of protein;
peanut butter and jelly sandwich (2 whole wheat slices)—16 g of protein
peanut butter and hummus (2 whole wheat slices)—19 g of protein
  (a personal favorite)
8-oz 1% milk—8 g protein
5.3-oz Dannon® Oikos® Greek yogurt (or comparable yogurt)—15 g of protein
4-tbsp hummus—3 g of protein—disappointing!
6 small 2.25-in falafel patties (100 g)—13.5 g of protein
25 g of dry whey protein (bulk) (often added to a fruit smoothie, etc.)
3-oz soft Tofu—6.5 g of protein; 3.2 g fat

Summary

Classic diets are abnormal deviations from the food you normally consume and they are usually difficult to stay on. It is much better to change your basic lifestyle in order to keep from becoming heavier. This includes learning how to cook, joining a food coop, and structuring your commute to work or school so that you walk a significant part of the way and also climb stairs and relax as you are waiting at various points during the commute. Going to a moderately lower-carbohydrate diet can be done by training oneself to cut down a little on carbohydrates. This can be done most effectively by using a ceremonial bowl for your principal whole starch eaten at meal times (rice, pasta, even bread). At the same time, it is relatively easy to nudge your protein in the diet higher by 5% of Calories (up to 21% of total Calories). It requires you to choose from the many high-protein foods now available.

Some Recent Studies that Have Reinforced My Thinking on the Obesity Explosion

Is There Something Special about Classic Low-Carbohydrate Diets?
Are Low-Carbohydrate Diets the Best Way to Lose Weight?

Yes, there is something special about low-carbohydrate diets. Since carbohydrates have provided, and still provide, a majority of Calories in most diets, eating a low-carbohydrate diet will decrease the amount of Calories consumed. That's how low-carbohydrate diets work. Are low-carbohydrate diets the best way to lose weight? No, many studies have confirmed that a low-carbohydrate diet is not better than other diets to lose weight.

But the most important question is, "Is eating a low-carbohydrate diet a reasonable and healthy way to live your life every day?" Since the main sources of complex carbohydrates, the principal starches, contain important components of the diet, including fiber and a whole spectrum of nutrients, that answer is probably no. And epidemiological studies bear this out. In a short-term study,[1] when a very low carbohydrate diet (<30 grams of carbohydrates per day) was served to patients for 14 days, there were several improvements in metabolic parameters, including decreased liver de novo fat synthesis and increased vitamin folate in the blood. However, in a long-term study,[2] where 15,428 adults, aged 45 to 64 years, who were

---

[1] Mardinoglu A, Wu H, Bjornson EB, Zhang C, Hakkarainen A, Räsänen SM, Lee S, Mancina RM, Bergentall M, Pietiläinen KH, Söderlund S, Matikainen N, Ståhlman M, Bergh P-O, Adiels M, Piening BD, Granér M, Lundbom N, Williams KJ, Romeo S, Nielsen J, Snyder M, Uhlén M, Bergström G, Perkins R, Marschall H-U, Bäckhed F, Taskinen M-R, Borén J (2018). An integrated understanding of the rapid metabolic benefits of a carbohydrate-restricted diet on hepatic steatosis in humans. *Cell Metabol* 27(3): 559–571. https://www.ncbi.nlm.nih.gov/pmc/?term=6706084

[2] Seidelmann SB, Claggett B, Cheng S, Henglin M, Shah A, Steffen LM, Folsom AR, Rimm EB, Willett WC, Solomon SD (2018). Dietary carbohydrate intake and mortality: a prospective cohort study and meta-analysis. *Lancet Public Health* 3(9): e419–e428. https://pubmed.ncbi.nlm.nih.gov/30122560

enrolled in the years 1987–1989 in the Atherosclerosis Risk in Communities (ARIC) study, an association was found between a low-carbohydrate diet and increased mortality. This observation has been seen in several large scale epidemiology studies. Therefore, there is great concern about the healthiness of consuming a very–low-carbohydrate diet in the long term.

Let's address the question of whether Classic low-carbohydrate diets are the best and easiest way to lose weight. The myth of the magic weight loss–promoting effects of the classic low-carbohydrate diet has been addressed by trained nutritionists over many years. However, for some reason, this myth has persisted, and may have recently gained more traction due to unsubstantiated reports on social media and the Internet.

Two recent studies involving meta-analysis (a type of statistical analysis that compares different studies that have similarities in experimental design) of the available, highly controlled dietary experiments have hopefully put to bed the notion that Classic low-carbohydrate diets have some magic ability to lead to weight loss.

I will review these recent studies to let you know the most recent research. As you will see, the findings were similar to what has been observed many times before. The first study[3] was published by Drs. Kevin Hall and J Guo from the National Institutes of Health in Bethesda, Maryland. The study involved a meta-analysis of 32 published studies that specifically investigated the effects of the level of carbohydrate in isocaloric diets (i.e., diets containing the same kilocalories per day) on energy expended and body fat accumulation. The results of Dr. Hall and Dr. Guo's meta-analysis indicated that a majority of the included studies showed that a subject's energy expenditure was greater when they consumed low-fat diets. What this means is that their metabolism did not mysteriously lower because they were eating the low-fat diet. This observation alone was an important finding because it countered a major argument put forth by "low-carbohydrate" enthusiasts. The meta-analysis also showed that lower-fat diets fostered greater body fat loss (as opposed to weight, which includes lean mass, water, and fat mass). Therefore, across many studies performed over a long period of time, a Classic low-carbohydrate diet, which in fact, is a high-fat diet, was not better for weight loss. The authors commented that "In other words, for all practical purposes 'a calorie is a calorie' when it comes to body fat and energy expenditure differences between controlled isocaloric diets varying in the ratio of carbohydrate to fat."

---

[3] Hall KD, Guo J (2017). Obesity energetics: Body weight regulation and the effects of diet composition. *Gastroenterology* 152(7): 1718–1727. https://www.ncbi.nlm.nih.gov/pubmed/28193517

The idea that a low-carbohydrate diet is better for weight loss than other diets has been disproven many times over the past 40 years.

I often say in my class that when two major studies essentially come up with the same data and conclusions, then one can have more confidence in both studies. This is exactly what happened in this case, although the second study asked slightly different questions. The second study by Sartorius et al. also used the meta-analysis method (i.e., comparing many published studies with reasonably similar protocols).[4] They concluded that a high-carbohydrate diet per se did not lead to obesity, nor did a diet with a high percentage of Calories coming from carbohydrate predispose a person toward obesity. The authors of this meta-analysis commented, "Based on our findings it cannot be concluded that a high-carbohydrate diet, or increased percentage of total energy intake in the form of carbohydrates, increases the odds of being obese. Mounting evidence exists, however, to indicate that the obesity epidemic has occurred during the industrial food era that has promoted the increased intake of refined carbohydrates and sugars." Therefore, both studies, the one by Kevin Hall and J. Guo, and the study by Sartorius et al., using the meta-analysis method, came to the same conclusions concerning Classic low-carbohydrate diets and weight loss. The definite conclusion was that a Classic low-carbohydrate diet does not convey any magical properties that make it better for weight loss.

The above two referenced studies used the meta-analysis method. Essentially, they are reviews of other studies, and they are not direct clinical intervention trials that recruit and study human subjects. Since questions still remain about what causes obesity and what might be the best way to treat obesity, additional clinical trial with different diets are continuing. In February 2018, Dr. Christopher Gardner's research group at Stanford University conducted a direct diet intervention, randomized controlled trial (called DIETFITS) to test whether a certain genotype pattern, or predetermined basic insulin secretion sensitivity, was associated with whether a Classic low-carbohydrate or a Classic low-fat diet was better for weight loss.[5]

---

[4] Sartorius K, Sartorius B, Madiba TE, Stefan C (2018). Does high-carbohydrate intake lead to increased risk of obesity? A systematic review and meta-analysis. *BMJ Open* 8(2):e018449. https://www.ncbi.nlm.nih.gov/pubmed/29439068

[5] Gardner CD, Trepanowski JF, Del Gobbo LC, Hauser ME, Rigdon J, Ioannidis JPA, Desai M, King AC (2018). Effect of low-fat vs low-carbohydrate diet on 12-month weight loss in overweight adults and the association with genotype Pattern or Insulin Secretion: The DIETFITS Randomized Clinical Trial. *JAMA* 319(7): 667–679. https://www.ncbi.nlm.nih.gov/pubmed/29466592

About 600 adults were recruited to eat either a healthy low-fat diet or a healthy low-carbohydrate diet for a 1-year period. In each group, 79% of the adults completed the 12-month study. Each group received extensive counseling on how to stay on their respective diets. After 1 year, the results of consuming the different diets on weight loss and on metabolic parameters were clear. "In this 12-month weight-loss diet study, there was no significant difference in weight change between a healthy low-fat diet versus a healthy low-carbohydrate diet, and neither genotype pattern nor baseline insulin secretion was associated with the dietary effects on weight loss. In the context of these two common weight-loss diet approaches, neither of the two hypothesized predisposing factors was helpful in identifying which diet was better for whom." This is now considered a "gold standard" trial in testing the utility of Classic low-carbohydrate diets for weight loss and health. As in many previous studies, there was no difference as to which diet was better for weight loss, and the results did not appear to involve basic insulin secretion. Interestingly, eating healthy in the Stanford study caused each group of subjects, on average, to lower their Calorie intake by a similar extent over the course of the study, leading to comparable weight losses.

There happened to be an important finding in the Stanford study that was brewing just below the surface of the study. Studies done up until now may have missed something that is an important factor in determining whether a diet works. And certainly each human that enrolls in a clinical trial is incredibly complex, and many issues that could interfere with a large study of this type may come into play and negate the impact of what is being studied in the first place. This is not to say that the factor being tested (in this case level of macronutrients) is not an important factor. It is just saying that other factors in play in the lives of free-living humans have additional influences that may mask the original question being asked.

An Investigative Reporter Gets to the Core of the DIETFITS Randomized Clinical Trial

Although the main results of the Stanford study were crystal clear, there were some very interesting data that came out of this study. In their article published in the prestigious Journal of the American Medical Association (JAMA), the authors included, albeit in the supplementary materials, a graph called a waterfall plot, that showed the distribution of responses for every subject in both groups of the study. This graph is shown below:

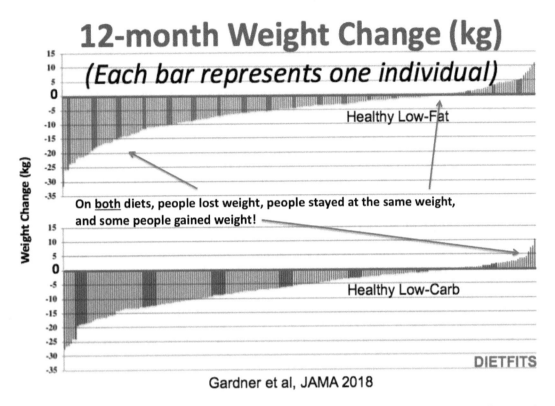

Gardner et al, JAMA 2018

This graph is from the Supplementary Materials addendum to the DietFits study conducted at Stanford University by Dr. Christopher Gardner et al. JAMA. 2018:319(7):667–679. Each vertical bar of different shading represents the results of one subject in the trial. This is an updated figure sent to the author by Dr. Gardner.

In addition to the average weight loss being similar between the low-carbohydrate and low-fat diet groups, the range of responses were also similar. On both diets, some of the subjects lost weight, some retained their weight, and some gained weight. What this means is that some factor, or group of factors, outside the design of the study was having a dominant effect on the overall responses of the humans being studied.

Julia Bulluz, an investigative health reporter for Vox media, asked permission to interview some of the subjects who were in the study.[6] She ended up interviewing two subjects who lost a significant amount of weight, and two subjects who did not lose weight.

---

[6] https://www.vox.com/science-and-health/2018/3/13/17054146/diet-isnt-working-why

Although she interviewed only a small number of the participants from the Stanford study, the subjects who were interviewed show how complex humans are and how outside forces can interfere with one's pursuit of health. In the two subjects who lost a great deal of weight after 1 year (one on the low-carbohydrate, and one on the low-fat diet), there were other factors present that motivated them to lose weight, and to change their lifestyles to eat and live healthier. One subject, spurred on by wanting to be healthier for his children, changed jobs so he could walk 2 miles to work and 2 miles back from work every day, whereas previously he drove hours a day on crowded California highways to go and return from work. Additionally, he gave up drinking alcohol and had more time to cook healthier foods at home. The other successful subject was a woman whose sister was recently diagnosed with cancer. She basically changed her lifestyle because of this wake up call, and she also wanted to show a good example for her children, who were starting to fall into unhealthy eating habits. Both of these participants made major changes in their lives, and the result was that they became healthier and also lost weight.

In the two subjects who did not lose weight after 1 year in the study (again one was on the low-carbohydrate diet and one was on the low-fat diet), the interfering factors were more nebulous and harder to describe. The woman who ate the low-carbohydrate diet found it difficult to fit exercise into her busy daily routine. Although she followed the directions of the low-carbohydrate diet, she substituted healthy but high-caloric, high-fat foods for the high-carbohydrate foods that she normally ate. Therefore, her Calorie intake on the low-carbohydrate diet did not drop, and the results were that she did not lose weight. The man who did not lose weight on the low-fat diet still remained in his very–low-movement job (sitting at a desk in front of a computer all day or driving for long hours in congestive traffic to branch offices). He still ate high-fat and high-calorie snacks and fast food along the road, and he did not put time or energy into living a healthy life.

The results from this mini-investigation have been hypothesized by researchers for many years. In order to be successful to maintain a healthy weight, a person has to change their lifestyle to one that is healthier. Long-term improvements in weight should not even be the first concern. And above all, both motivation and adequate time and resources are needed to be able to take care of yourself and the members of your family.

These three studies, the first two of which reviewed many previous studies that tested the effects of carbohydrate level in the diet on weight loss, and the third, a well-designed clinical intervention trial, all came to the same conclusion—the actual macronutrient makeup of the diet is not a significant factor per se in whether a diet is effective or not. What determines the effectiveness of these diets, and really any diet, is how you nudge yourself closer to a healthy lifestyle, and whether you have the resources to commit time and finances to being healthy.

What Is It with Processed Foods? Why Do They Influence Food Intake?

What is it about ultraprocessed foods that make them candidates for being involved in the Obesity Explosion? We really do not know. In fact, until recently, there has never been a randomized clinical trial that tested the beneficial effects of reducing ultraprocessed foods in the diet. However a study was published in 2018 that was the first randomized clinical trial to test this hypothesis.

Dr. Kevin Hall's research group at the National Institutes of Health in Bethesda, Maryland, published a study[7] that tested the concept that people eating a diet containing mostly low-processed foods would lead to a lower-calorie intake than if the same people ate an isocaloric diet of ultraprocessed foods. The reasoning behind doing this clinical trial was the hypothesis that there is something unique about ultraprocessed foods that causes increased consumption of Calories. Possible unique qualities are that they bypass normal food intake regulatory mechanisms, or that their intrinsic greater energy density leads to increased Calorie intake.

Twenty subjects (mean age 31 and mean BMI of 27) were recruited to consume, ad libitum, either an ultraprocessed diet or a low-processed diet for 14 days. After consuming one of the diets, the subjects crossed-over to eat the other diet for 14 days. Each subject consumed each of the diets in a metabolic ward at the NIH during the entire length of the study. The diets, as presented to the subjects, contained similar amounts of Calories, sugar, fat, fiber, and macronutrients. The subjects had an hour to eat each meal after it was presented to them. Each day there was a different distinctly set of meals, and the daily menus were rotated on a 7-day schedule. Intakes of food and Calories were measured for each diet, and the results showed that subjects who ate the ultraprocessed diet consumed an average of about 500 more kcal/day than the people eating the low-processed diet. Furthermore, their body weights reacted in a predictable way in that the subjects either maintained or increased their weight over the subjects eating the low-processed diet, who for the most part lost weight.

Over the course of 14 days, the average intake of Calories was increased when the ultraprocessed diets were consumed compared to when the unprocessed diets were consumed. The increases were apparent on the first day of consuming the diets and

---

[7] Hall KD, Ayuketah A, Brychta R, Cai H, Cassimatis T, Chen KY, Chung ST, Costa E, Courville A, Darcey V, Fletcher LA, Forde CG, Gharib AM, Guo J, Howard R, Joseph PV, McGehee S, Ouwerkerk R, Raisinger K, Rozga I, Stagliano M, Walter M, Walter PJ, Yang S, Zhou M (2019). Ultra-processed diets cause excess calorie intake and weight gain: An inpatient randomized controlled trial of ad libitum food intake. *Cell Metabol* 30(1): 226. doi: 10.1016/j.cmet.2019.05.020. PMID: 31269427 https://www.ncbi.nlm.nih.gov/pubmed/?term=31269427

they were carried through the entire 14-day period. The ultraprocessed group consumed about 3,000 kcal/day, whereas the group eating unprocessed food consumed about 2,500 kcal/day. Carbohydrate (280 ± 54 kcal/day; $p < 0.0001$) and fat (230 ± 53 kcal/day; $p = 0.0004$) intakes were both higher in the people eating the ultraprocessed diets. Since the meals that were presented to each group were matched for macronutrients, fiber, total Calories, energy density, sugar, and sodium, some other difference must have affected the consumption of these foods.

What do ultraprocessed foods have that may spur humans on to increase their intake of Calories?

Some of the candidates include flavorings, the composition of the fats, potassium, and the ratio of refined to unrefined grains. Concerning the equivalent fiber contents of the diets, whole grains have many more nutrients then refined grains besides fiber.

As far as palatability was concerned, there were no complaints that the low-processed diet was less pleasant or satisfying than the ultraprocessed diet.

In real life, ultraprocessed foods are often more energy dense than low-processed foods. In the Hall NIH study, this was not the case as both diets were made purposely the same caloric density. The difference in Calorie intake occurred when the subjects ate more of the presented meal.

Concerning other differences that there may have been between the diets, photos of all the meal used in this study were included in the supplementary material (Go to the journal article to see photos of the meals).

Looking at the photos of the prepared meals, when you go rapidly back and forth through them, what hit me first was that the unprocessed foods were a lot greener—especially the lunches and dinners. So I am wondering, could there be the differences in beta carotene and other carotenoids and flavonoids between the diets? Also, I wonder if it may be the potassium and vitamin K contents of the unprocessed foods versus the processed foods. The sodium amounts were the same, but the potassium had to be greater in the diets comprised of unprocessed food, I would think.

Also, since the unprocessed food required more chewing, could it be that time and energy put into chewing made a difference? Is there a chewing sensor?

Also, the unprocessed diet was lower in saturated fat and higher in both omega-3 and omega-6 fatty acids. Could this have been a major difference?

The overall conclusions from this last article were that minimally processed foods lead to lower-calorie intake. The authors commented, tongue in cheek I suppose, that this conclusion could provide additional problems as adhering to a diet with mainly low-processed foods requires more time and skill to prepare these foods.

Summary of the Obesity Explosion

The major theme of this book is that unless you know the causes of the Obesity Explosion, you will not know how to combat it. This applies to both the country and the individual. As an individual, you have to be able to tell the difference between what is true and what is hype concerning nutrition. After reading this book, I hope you will have the knowledge to differentiate between all the noise that comes from the Internet nutrition experts and what is actually accurate information. When you feel deeply that you are on the correct path to healthy living, you won't fall for the quack Classic diet books that are out there.

The one stunning observation in this book that towers above all the others is that just a small increase in intake of 50 to 300 kcal/day above a person's total daily energy expenditure will cause most of us to gain weight. If this is carried forward for many years, people can become significantly obese. Through 10,000 years of agriculture, our bodies have done a fine job keeping us a certain weight. The discovery that such a small increase in intake can lead to such a large weight increase can only mean that most of us have an extraordinary, sensitive system that regulates daily food intake, and that it has only been in the past 50 years where enough changes were made in our world such that this system became overwhelmed. In teaching a course in Nutrition for over 28 years, I have often thought that the following factors are the ones that have had the greatest effects on overruling the masterful human food intake regulation system:

1. In most communities today, food is available all around us for the entire year. For most of humanity, there was a portion of the year, usually due to climate, when food was scarce at particular times due to winter or to an extremely dry period.

2. There are now thousands of different foods available, and it is easy to find something in a mega supermarket that appeals to your taste on any particular day.

3. Processed foods have a quality about them that spurs over consumption (detailed in Chapter 17). It may be that they contain special flavors, it may be a precise ratio of salt, sugar, and fat, or it may be that they are more Calorie dense.

These three factors, when joined by a constellation of other factors discussed throughout this book, have made it extremely difficult for a large percentage of our population to remain at a healthier weight.

Another major point in this book is that Classic diets do not work. The reasons may be obscure, but my bet is that it is because they are artificial and not natural. Any diet that tries to alter the basic amounts of macronutrients extremely and artificially is bound to fail for most people.

So the question becomes, what is a person to do?

Now that the factors have been laid out in this book, this is up to every individual to decide for himself or herself.

A logical path would be to reverse everything that happened nutritionally and energy engaging over the past 50 to 100 years. Here are my thoughts on this:

On the Cultural, Political and Economic Level:

1. Avoid processed foods and commit the time and effort to shop for healthy foods in a small market or food co-op. Nationally, food co-ops, especially those that sell directly from farmers, should be given tax-free status. Food assistance should go twice as far in these small, healthy markets.
2. Having the time and ability to shop for healthy foods can only be accomplished for most people if the economic system was adjusted so that people had enough nonworking time and resources to pursue shopping and eating healthy.
3. The Physical-Built environment should be structured to be healthier with cleaner air, safe and environmentally friendly transportation, and recreation areas that are convenient, large and safe for everyone.

On the Nutritional Level:

Nutritionally follow a diet that resembles and has the main components of the Mediterranean Diet, as this diet and lifestyle has been shown historically, and through clinic trials, to be the healthiest diet. The main components of this diet are:

a) Reliance on principal starches that are not highly processed and contain their most of their original fiber and nutrients.
b) Consumption of a wide variety of green vegetables
c) Low intake of meat
d) Use of fats that have high monounsaturated fats (olive oil) and high omega-3 fatty acid food products (canola oil, flax seed, nuts, and marine foods). There should only be a small amount of other vegetable oils, such as soybean oil, in the diet
e) Exposure to moderate sunshine throughout the year

On a Personal Level:

This is the area that each of us has to determine based upon our own life experiences. The nonnutritional factors that have influenced the Obesity Explosion that I have written about in this book are not the only ones. There are probably dozens more. Any factor that lowers a person's daily activity level (also known as NEAT) should be countered. Jim Levine's research, and studies on the effects of television viewing, have basically indicated that, on average, Americans are less active by about 2 to 2.5 hours/day than we were before all the energy influencing devices were invented and implemented during the 20th century. Therefore, each of us needs to increase our daily energy expending activities by about 2 hours/day.

It is this simple, and that difficult.

Joseph L. Dixon grew up in Brooklyn, NY, and attended Brooklyn Prep High School and later the State University of New York at Binghamton. He received M.S. and Ph.D. degrees in Nutritional Sciences from the University of Wisconsin-Madison. In 1983, he went to Columbia University for post-doctoral research on Vitamin A metabolism. After a research position at the New York Blood Center, he returned to Columbia University to study fat, cholesterol and lipoproteins. In 2004, he moved to Rutgers University, New Jersey, which has a strong lipid research group. Dr. Dixon is a lipid biochemist, cell biologist, and an Associate Professor of Nutritional Sciences in the Department of Nutritional Sciences at Rutgers University, New Brunswick, NJ. He has been teaching courses on Nutrition, including a course entitled, Nutrition and Health, for over 25 years. His specific research interests are lipid and cholesterol metabolism and the mass spectrometry of lipids. His other books can be viewed on his website, http://www.josephldixon.com

ACKNOWLEDGMENTS

Acknowledgments for the Obesity Explosion

This book was made a hundred times better by the many reviewers who helped by spending their valuable time reviewing early chapters and later versions for this book and having valuable discussions concerning obesity and health. I especially would like to thank the following: Henry Blackburn, M.D., Mayo Professor Emeritus of the University of Minnesota; Anita Brinker, Ph.D., Environmental and Occupational Health Sciences Institute, Rutgers University, NJ; Carol Byrd-Bredbenner, Ph.D., R.D., Professor of the Department of Nutritional Sciences, Rutgers University, NJ; Hans Fisher, Ph.D., Emeritus Professor of Nutritional Sciences, Rutgers University, NJ; James A. Levine, M.D., Ph.D., Professor, Mayo Clinic and Arizona State University: Curtis W. Marean, Ph.D., Foundation Professor, School of Human Evolution and Social Change, Arizona State University; Charlotte N. Markey, Ph.D., Professor of Psychology, Rutgers University, NJ; Joshua W. Miller, Ph.D., Professor of Nutritional Sciences, Rutgers University, NJ; Robert H Miller, Ph.D., Lyons, CO, retired Vice President and Global Head of Nutrition Research at Abbott Labs; Debra Palmer Keenan, Ph.D., M.Ed., Associate Professor of Nutritional Sciences, Rutgers University, NJ; NJ State Coordinator for the Expanded Food and Nutrition Education Program (EFNEP); and, former NJ Director, Supplemental Nutrition Assistance Program Education (SNAP-Ed); Daniel H. Sandweiss, Ph.D., Professor of Anthropology and Director, School of Policy and International Affairs, University of Maine; Sue Shapses, Ph.D., R.D., Professor of Nutritional Sciences, Rutgers University, NJ; Joanne Slavin, Ph.D., R.D., Professor of Nutrition, Department of Nutritional Sciences, University of Minnesota; Judith Storch, Ph.D., R.D.; Distinguished Professor of Nutritional Sciences, Rutgers University, NJ; Malcolm Watford, D.Phil., Professor of Nutritional Sciences, Rutgers University, NJ; John Worobey, Ph.D., Professor of Nutritional Sciences, Rutgers University, NJ.

Thank you to the following researchers for providing original artwork from their publications: George A. Brooks, Ph.D., Professor of Integrative Biology, University of California, Berkley; Steven Heymsfield, M.D., Professor, Pennington Biomedical Research Center, Baton Rouge, LA; Christopher Gardner, Ph.D., Rehnborg Farquhar Professor, Stanford University.

I would like to thank the thousands of students (over two thousand since Spring 2017 alone) who were in my class, Nutrition and Health, at Rutgers University. Many commented on early versions of the chapters in this book. They also inspired me to write it!

I especially thank Roberta Kopp, M.A., who pre-edited the entire book and helped with its structure and design. Thank you to acquisition editor, Sue Saad, and project coordinator, Joshua La Rue, of Kendall-Hunt, who shepherded the book through final editing and production.